FACING SURGERY?
DON'T BE A SCAREDY CAT

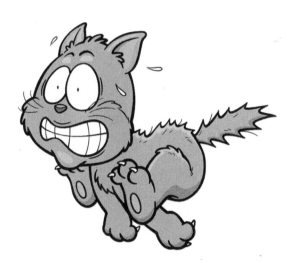

FACING SURGERY?
DON'T BE A SCAREDY CAT

BY

ALAN CHARNLEY

Contents

DON'T SHOOT THE MESSENGER

First, this book is dedicated to those of you who might be about to go into hospital for surgery and who may feel afraid. I hope it gives you encouragement as well as a few tips to alleviate your worries and beat the stress of it all.

It is also dedicated to those of us adults who since childhood have been afraid to seek medical treatment or go for health check-ups because we suffer from *White Coat Syndrome* – anxiety around for instance doctors or nurses or prompted when we visit surgeries or hospitals. Just the sight or smell of anything remotely medical sends our blood pressure soaring.

This book too is a nudge for you to get yourself checked for cancer, or for that matter any other condition if you feel poorly and have symptoms that concern you, not do as I did and leave it until the outcome or prognosis is far worse...

This book is also the story of the loss of my father who died from cancer – radiation poisoning – after going to Nagasaki in Japan in 1946 to clean up after the American's dropped their atomic bomb. I ask, is my cancer hereditary and the result of that bomb?

I also write about my long-term associations with journalism and pop music because I hope you'll find the anecdotes amusing and I can name drop.

And what about gender and sexuality these days? Hear it from someone who is pleased that in these modern times there are new labels that identify those of us who might have thought ourselves, before the arrival of them into the vocabulary, to be outsiders making up forgotten or neglected minorities.

With current inclusivity and embracing of minorities as well as our ongoing developing vocabulary for dialogue, then with a little more patience, discussion, understanding and go-ahead thinking amongst us all, then at whatever age we are or reach, it should not be necessary for some to hide away or feel alone in the world for gender, race or belief issues.

Finally, and most engagingly, Facebook – now calling itself Meta – gets a bad press at times, but my story tells how a 91-year-old mother, Gladys Judith Charnley, re-united with her 67-year-old son Alan – your truly – after a 50-year plus estrangement. Our reunion started and continued by messaging one another on that social network and some 80,000 words were exchanged. We met just the once shortly before her death. You couldn't make up such a strange story and I haven't!

When I began writing about my encounter with cancer, I didn't know where to stop so it turned into a little bit of a pocket autobiography! I was dipping my toe in the water writing this and therefore it represents only a small slice of my life, mainly the unusual beginnings. That has meant many of those I love dearly and are important to me and stood by me when I was diagnosed with cancer are not name checked but you know who you are and how much I value the love and support you have shown me.

But first let's deal with the health check averse scaredy cats. I used to be one so if you're out there and reading this then I know how you feel.

As I did, you too can beat white coat syndrome…

CHAPTER ONE

OWN GOAL

Using a football analogy, I had scored the stupidest of own goals – and after the removal of two cancer tumours in a major operation lasting eight hours that also involved a blood transfusion, cancer could even now still cost me my life.

It still hasn't gone away completely. I am being monitored.

During my time spent working for Cancer Research UK, the UK's biggest cancer charity in Britain, as a regional media officer I spent long hours writing and mailing thousands of media releases urging people to get tested if they experienced cancer symptoms. The earlier you presented yourself to doctors I preached to the population of this country the greater your chances of survival. I worked hard and was devout to the cause and I hope by my efforts as a messenger I helped save a few lives along the way.

But my secret was that while delivering that sensible cancer message urging the public to respond to their possible cancer symptoms and to get themselves tested, I personally ignored the charity's advice because I suffered from 'white coat syndrome'.

I was fearful of treatment because I had a dread of visiting hospitals or doctor's surgeries. This 'fear' dated back to my childhood.

My own cancer diagnosis came in my seventh decade – and sure enough because for a significant time I had ignored tell-tale symptoms that something was wrong with me, my outcome was worse, much worse.

It led to major surgery – the eight-hour operation and a blood transfusion to save my life. I, now also live with a stoma.

The reason for this book is to encourage you get yourself tested!

Yes – here's that message again – if you have tell-tale symptoms that something is wrong with your health get yourself checked out. Now!

Also now, this scaredy cat having gone through gruelling treatment, can offer advice to others like himself. If you're a scaredy cat too facing surgery or treatment for cancer or going 'under the knife' for any other procedure, my latest advice also includes this message – no need to be scared, just go ahead with the surgery or prescribed treatment and don't whatever you do 'overthink' it beforehand!

In my days working for CRUK and before that Cancer Research Campaign, I interviewed hundreds of cancer patients. Some of these men and women survived following advanced and latest treatments being offered to ensure their survival but others less fortunate had to accept that nothing could be done for them. Many of the unfortunate ones, but not all by any means, presented themselves too late for treatment to save their lives.

I must have distributed thousands of stories to national and regional media. I went on radio and TV spreading the message – do it, don't delay get yourself tested. That was the mantra.

I recruited TV stars who were willing to endorse that message. There was for instance actor Julie Hesmondhalgh, who playing popular trans character Hayley on Coronation Street and Tony Audenshaw, the cheerful and chirpy Bob from ITV's soap Emmerdale. Both especially kind and lovely people who helped along the way.

Mind you, I did once engage the BBC football match commentator who had long since starred on TV's *It's a Knockout*. How was I to know Stuart Hall would end up in jail later for sordid sex crimes? He was good at what he did for me on that day I had innocently recruited him as a volunteer to wear a boxing glove – 'Let's Knockout Cancer' – was the punchline of the story promoting the research work of the Paterson Institute, the scientific arm of the Christie Hospital in Manchester.

As a fit bloke who had run or walked everywhere during his seven decades on planet earth I revelled in my fitness. But unbeknown to anyone else I was behaving like an ostrich with its head in the sand. I had experienced spells of feeling strangely unwell. My jogging was slowing too. My health seemed to be deteriorating and looking back in the mirror a drawn face stared back at me, considerably thinner than it used to be.

However, like a lot of people, but especially men, I ignored these signals. My health would improve naturally on its own. These sorts of twinges and bouts of unwellness happened but always passed. They had before, honest! There was another factor holding me back too – I never did like to make a fuss about what could turn out to be nothing.

Then one night at home sat on the sofa I left it briefly to brew a cuppa and returned to find it covered in blood. I couldn't ignore that, even if I believed myself to be a scaredy cat too when it came to seeking medical treatment.

The seeds of my aversion to doctors and nurses were sewn in my childhood. This was the start of my white coat syndrome. The sight of a needle would send me cold with fear. Would my heart stop beating if the doctor put a stethoscope to my chest? If my blood pressure was taken the squeezing tight of a tourniquet on my arm sent my heartbeat off the scale leaving it pounding in my chest. One adult reading of my blood pressure at one hospital caused a nurse to say: "That can't be right you should be dead. It must be the machine."

More likely I thought the reading was greatly enhanced by my fearful fight or flight responses.

Since a child and into adulthood, I never did have the courage to visit a dentist. They always wore white coats.

The first time I did visit one, aged about nine accompanied by my mother, I had experienced what I supposed to be the worst nightmare ever known to a child. I was riding on a superfast, high roller coaster ride. The dentist had put me under with gas. I awoke from my nightmare as my head crashed through the metal track at the end of the ride. My head was smashing through metal and that was my awakening from that nightmare. It has stayed vivid in my memory to this day.

Suffering mind-numbing toothache once more aged about 20, I plucked up the courage to visit another dentist but having my teeth drilled for fillings proved an equally horrendous second experience and I absented once more from future treatment.

I had met strange doctors too on the occasions when I was either taken by my mother to a surgery as a child or was so desperate to attend as an adult, I bit a bullet and dragged myself there once or twice.

Aged around five I suffered terrifying nightmares, and this was before my visit to Mr Dread the Dentist and his knock-out gas. As a child I used to fear the fall of night and dropping asleep because the same nightmare always haunted me. I had no way of explaining what it was that was happening to me, but it was a nightmare scenario. Indescribable as it was terrifying.

The more I think about it in later life the only sense I make of it is that it might have been a memory of being inside the womb. I was in a gaseous confined place and there was pumping and hissing. Experts are sceptical of this occurring however other people report it too. I can only state what I believe might be the case. The question is how far back in the foetal development process does the brain recall?

Anyway, my mother was sufficiently concerned to inform a doctor about my nightmares, and when we arrived at his surgery, he did what all doctors do, the answer to everything doctors did I used to think, he sounded my chest!

Stood there in my vest, I recall his disdain at having to bother with me as well having this overwhelming feeling that he thought I was lying. He asked me one or two abrupt, snappy questions and then concluded like a crabby schoolmaster to my mother: "There's nothing wrong with this boy."

My mother and I were packed off. The nightmares continued until I grew a little older and then they did eventually fade without me ever knowing why I experienced them in the first place or any significance.

Another 'White Coat' experience that I experienced as a child, and I remember vividly, were my regular visits to The Chest Clinic which I was obliged to attend as a preventative measure.

Yes, it was for my own good, I was told. But in later years as an adult try explaining to others the most bizarre thing you did as a child. Most of my peers couldn't believe it when I told them that kids with suspected weak chests like me in the late 50's and early 60's were sent to sit facing a huge bright lamp in the centre of a room. When I did tell anyone they either (a) believed I'd told them a big fat lie or (b) that I was trying to tell them that as a kid I was abducted by aliens.

My mother because of her TB and to boost the health of her damaged lungs took me fortnightly to a room in Gainsborough, Lincolnshire, the town where we lived at the time. That room if my memory serves me well, may well have been attached to a place I dreaded, a doctor's surgery or a hospital. I do remember the staff all wore those scary white coats.

In this large room where around 20 people gathered for each session, we were confronted by a machine centred in the room that threw out a brilliant bright, dazzling light. This was a Sunray Machine, and its recipients were mainly mothers sat around on a circle of chairs with their offspring suitably prepared by being bare chested or wearing string vests.

We all wore green goggles so that our eyes would not be damaged, these goggles made the entire room appear green. You could imagine you were underwater in a deep green murky seaweed strewn sea. If Paul McCartney's Frog Song had been around it would have made a fun soundtrack to this scenario. This was well before the advent of space travel films like Star Trek otherwise an alternative scenario would have been that we were indeed human sacrifices about to be beamed up by aliens. No wonder I never fancied attending medical appointments. White coat syndrome. People in white coats led us into that room.

Cancer experts are notorious for not knowing when we ask what precisely caused our cancers. We all are puzzled as to whether we contributed in some way to the disease. We'd like to know precisely where it was that we went wrong in our lives to cause it. Yes, they do know when the lungs are as black as coals it's a safe bet it's probably the fags that have been responsible. And now with the benefit of hindsight the Sunray treatment that I went for as a child in the late 50's early 60's is considered unsafe. That then was rather the equivalent of sun seekers these days staying far too long under sun beds.

We were being fried for our own good.

Some specialists are convinced that this childhood sunray treatment is the cause of skin cancers in adults treated in this era.

Some physicians at the time were calling for regulation of these Sunray lamps, but they were so popular that most doctors ignored the possibility there could be long term safety concerns.

One reputable medic stated: "It is possible that late-onset skin cancers could be connected to childhood sunlamp treatment," but he carefully added "that one could never pinpoint the exact cause of such cancers."

A London dermatologist who sees hundreds of patients with skin cancers every year is convinced Sunray treatment could be linked.

He is quoted as saying that while the effects of ultra-violet light therapy many years ago cannot be separated from exposure to sunshine over the intervening years, he believes UV treatment will be responsible for at least some of the cancers now being seen. "Those Sunray lamps could have contributed to someone's future skin cancer risk," he said categorically.

"The damage caused to the skin tends to have a 20 to 40-year 'latency period' which explains why these people are noticing skin cancers now," he added.

Sun lamps were invented in the 1900s and one of the first regular users was King George V, who famously received light treatment for the near-fatal pneumonia he suffered in 1928.

The practice only ended in the late Sixties when antibiotics became available to all who needed them, rendering light-treatment redundant.

There is no way of knowing how many Sunray Therapy children went on to get skin cancer, and how many may not have survived its most serious forms.

......

When I was in my 20's I was concerned about a cough I couldn't shake off. As a last resort I went into a doctor's surgery and there was the doc stood in a corner with his back to me. He was staring at the wall. He looked like the school dunce banished into a corner as a punishment.

He began asking me questions but never once did his eyes switch from the wall to me.

Only to write a prescription did he leave his corner. Then looking downwards, he swiftly wrote the prescription at his desk which he quickly passed to me and then I left without him having had sight of who he'd just diagnosed. He wouldn't have recognised me ten minutes later walking down the street.

I told the tale of this odd behaving doctor to others in my locality and discovered they had similar encounters with him.

I was told he suffered from crippling shyness.

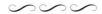

Possibly the doctor or was he a consultant with the worst bedside manner was the one examining me when – surprise, surprise – I did get my prostate checked and this was more than a decade before my recent cancer diagnosis.

Intolerable stomach pain forced me into that visit.

This medic was the spitting image of the bombastic on-screen actor James Robertson Justice, who often portrayed on films a gung-hospital consultant.

Of course, the necessary prostate examination is a rubber gloved finger up the bum. I don't envy any doctor who must perform this ritual week after week of his or her medical life, but 'James' was heavy handed to say the least.

He pushed and prodded and shouted at one stage: "Relax can't you. How can I do this if you're not relaxed."

There he stood, the most unrelaxed and aggressive doctor it had ever been my misfortune to encounter who had in his charge a sensitive soul like me and was handling me like a bag of spuds.

He told me after my examination that I now had to have blood samples taken from the prostate. I'd undergo that procedure at the hospital. I shuddered at the word hospital. I asked him if the procedure was painful.

"It'll be like being stung by a swarm of bees," he replied deadpan. Not a trace of humour. He's a sadist, I thought.

I later mentioned his behaviour to another doctor who was involved in the hospital testing itself, and he said: "Oh him. He's a law unto himself. I've heard similar stories about him from other patients."

I don't suppose anyone in authority did anything about this rogue creature. He was by then approaching retirement age anyway and I surmised wasn't about to change his ways for anyone. He was an old school physician doing precisely as he pleased to the discomfort and possible upset of many patients. He needed drumming out the NHS. Things thankfully seem to have changed a lot since those days…

And finally, what do you think when, as a child, nurses take away the Christmas presents Santa gave you to burn them?

Well, you might think you missed your proper turning and were being cared for by torturers, yet that was what happened to me.

Taken to an isolation hospital as an emergency with complications of chicken pox, I saw nothing but white coats and nurses for days when aged about 11 and given my own room.

I was given my presents on Christmas Day by the nurses but when I left my room more than a week later to go home, I was told the toys couldn't come with me because they were infectious and had to be incinerated.

CHAPTER TWO

MY CANCER DIAGNOSIS

My overall plan was to live out my natural and fit life and then suffer the consequences of not protecting my health much later. Then I hoped to die a quick and painless death and avoid needles, pills, surgery and the like… and now here I was finally facing the consequences of my philosophy with one question to answer. Did I want to continue living or to die?

Just before Christmas in December 2022 I was diagnosed with cancer.

Thud, crash, Ker pow! Shockwaves.

What will happen if I don't get treated, I tentatively asked the doctor at the hospital.

"It will kill you," she replied.

What I would say now to anyone facing treatment for cancer or any other disease is don't be a scaredy cat. If you must undergo radiotherapy, chemotherapy or surgery, bite the bullet and do it. Even if you THINK that you are the world's worst scaredy cat as I did, proceed with that treatment.

Focus on going through with it and follow the expert medical advice you will be offered – and you may just come out after treatment having surprised yourself by just how brave you are or can be.

Surprise yourself!

Once you've been through the treatment and are hopefully on the mend you may even self-diagnose your past thinking and behaviour as I have done. I reckon that I was often living in fear of the fear itself. Some of us are, you know. We overthink and fear the worst. If you have a lively imagination, as I have, it can lead you into dark places. If you're a hypochondriac too, you may immediately start thinking that if you are diagnosed with one malady, that other ailments are bound to follow in some bizarre domino effect.

Negativity may lead to you to asking what will go wrong when you have the treatment rather than what will go right.

These kind of over reactions or false trails will only lead you to stress and sleepless nights. Stop negative thinking in its tracks. Don't be tempted down these routes. If you recognise these sorts of thoughts creeping into your head – stop them immediately!

Everything can be plain sailing with your treatment should you allow it to be. Don't become your own worst enemy by fretting.

You'll never know how strong and resilient you are until you have had the courage to face your demons. Those demons might not be the treatment itself that you are facing, but instead how you deal with the irrational worries you may be having. You can best take care of yourself by not obsessing about what might happen or go wrong. What will happen, will happen and it is out of your control, but if your diagnosis is that you will survive a cancer, the experts have probably got it very right.

Too many patients probably needlessly overload themselves with unnecessary worry. Once you come out the other side, you may well own up to the fact that worrying became a bigger curse to you than the treatment itself, though some cancer patients will still argue and have just cause to do so that the treatment is worse than the disease itself, especially the often-nauseous effects of chemotherapy. I give my advice knowing that we all bring our differences of nature to the table. Advice isn't a one size fits all panacea – we all deal with treatment or the anticipation of it differently.

Yes, we are all different and process and deal with things in our own way, but I believe there can be nothing more helpful to new patients as hearing how others have successfully coped going through the same experiences as you are about to go through. These patients, who you can ask to meet or who you will be told about, will have been chosen wisely by medics of course and will have a positive outlook so they're highly unlikely to load upon you a negative horror story – and of course they'll be optimists, glass half full people with a smile upon their face and a 'there's nothing to it' attitude to treatment. Ask to meet one of these cheerful souls. Seek one out…

So here is how my cancer story began for me – this especially relevant to the scaredy cats amongst you in the hope that at least some of your fears may be allayed.

One autumn evening I stood up at home and saw my blood on my sofa, I rang the doctor's surgery early doors the very next day.

Okay though mine was an early call I found myself 19th in the queue and that was only to speak to the doctor's receptionist and oh what a bind it is these days waiting in such a long queue and having to listen to muzak that no-one in their right mind would choose to play to a patient like me, had they known of course that I can only tolerate decent music and not pap.

My first concern. Would I even get past the receptionist to see a doctor? How persuasive could I make my case? Isn't it a bit of a competition these days who gets seen and who doesn't? Is the patient who gets seen the one who can best explain the worst symptoms of their pain in the best and most expressive way or the noisiest act? Would I need to perform, show more emotion than usual, would I need to break down and sob for help? Did I need to produce an Oscar winning performance to be seen? Had you heard as I had one morning on radio and TV, to fill all would-be patients with gloom, that the UK's NHS was broken irreparably? Shudder.

What these days if you are horribly ill but too much of a bag of nerves to explain your condition on the phone? Will you miss out on an appointment because you are lacking communication skills? Tales abound these days of doctors not meeting worried patients or of some receptionists, not all of them mind you, behaving like Rottweilers and being difficult to bypass.

If I had listened to all the doubts that I have just listed and might have been swirling around my head at the time about making my call, I might have allowed this sad litany of excuses to win the day and not even bothered picking up my mobile phone.

Don't fall into that trap. Get on the phone. Persistence pays. Get on with it. You might even get a tune you like on their phone muzak system.

To my surgery's eternal credit, they saw me later that same day. I was given an appointment, and, in the afternoon, I arrived feeling pensive. The doc first checked I wasn't suffering from bleeding haemorrhoids. I wasn't and knew it instinctively too. Intuition was kicking in or could it have been hypochondria?

Two days after the doctor's examination, my home phone buzzed, and it was the hospital telling me to come in for an urgent colonoscopy at Stepping Hill Hospital, Stockport.

In the past I would have run a mile from this procedure. A camera up your bum is required for one of these. The fact I could no longer even run a mile in my condition to make my escape, made it a date imperative to keep. I liked being fit. I wanted to be fit again. I turned up. That's what you all should do, turn up. Life's winners are all people who just turned up.

That was the start of my new and positive mindset. I would be examined and do what I had to do. Tens of thousands of others had already been through these procedures and if they discovered something awful during my intimate body search, I would be offered helped with a treatment or be told otherwise. I might even have achieved peace of mind knowing all was well with my body or that they had diagnosed something as insignificant as severe indigestion.

If you fear the worst, as many of us do when facing these tests, you ask yourself – so what after this testing they should discover I only have a short time left to live!

Well, if you believe in life everlasting and God or like the Buddhists re-incarnation, then you may be happier at this stage than those that don't, but at this critical time maybe not THAT much happier. You may have a slight edge though over the agnostic or fatalist who believes that when we die 'that's our lot'.

Everlasting life means you can look forward to being reunited with those whom you have loved, those who you may miss and who have gone before you to prepare the way. They might even now be decorating, putting up spectacular baubles for your arrival in some celestial palace where the evening entertainment is a duet from Elvis Presley and Chuck Berry.

Cheer up. It may never happen. You are overthinking, especially if you think Elvis and Chuck are going to form a duo!

However, if you're a non-believer, the stark fact must be faced that we all die and we have a short life, though when we are younger, we think we may be immortal.

I think of it this way. In the great scheme of things, we're incredibly tiny things. Our life is smaller than a grain of sand, even less say than the size of an ant. The world managed without us for billions of years and will do so after we are gone.

But take further consolation from the fact that it might not be long before the entire human race follows you wherever you are going, by exterminating themselves in a pointless war. The planet will probably be destroyed by nuclear war. There can be advantage in dying sooner rather than later if trigger happy idiots use nuclear weapons. Trust me, that will be hell on earth and you're better off out of it.

Now after considering the end game and the possibility of enjoying a life everlasting, your next thoughts will turn to why you should try your level best to stay on earth for just a little while longer.

Most of us will start this process by making lists of perhaps (a) those people who might miss you if you leave too soon (b) unfinished business that you want to stay around too complete… Do you have a half-knitted jumper awaiting completion? Did you always intend to run a marathon? (c)Are there broken relationships in your life you would choose to repair if you are given a stay of execution?

All this thinking, most times premature, happens to us all at critical phases along life's passage, but especially when we're older or very ill.

Bucket lists may be compiled at an early stage of your diagnosis. It's time to produce a list of those things you promise yourself you will do and note these in the 'I Will Live' column on an A4 sheet of paper.

You can write why it will be so good to run that first marathon, finish knitting that jumper or raise money for the hospital treating you – on the understanding they do cure you.

You'll make deals with God. Please God save me, and I will never walk past a church again without calling in and donating. Don't worry if you can find nothing to scribble down under your other heading 'The Advantages of Dying'.

Throughout my dealing with the NHS, I have been immensely impressed by the fast-track procedure they lined up for me and

I am not a private patient who went to the front of the queue at the expense of others.

You can expect efficiency and TLC from medics and nurses.

When I was receiving treatment in the Radiotherapy Oncology Department and as I lay there being zapped, I realised how fortunate I was living in the United Kingdom with its National Health System compared to those people living in poorer countries. People who had the very same diagnosis as mine but had no access to what might prove to be lifesaving or very expensive treatment. Mind you, it was part of the deal I made with the Government. I did pay into the NHS all my working life. Now I didn't resent that fact that I had!

The NHS were fast to investigate and to diagnose. Very fast and efficient. Having said that you realise quickly that you have a responsibility to do your bit to make sure the course of treatment they have planned for you goes well.

Throughout my treatment process I was always early for appointments. I never postponed any of mine though I was informed that others did. Perhaps they were wanting to put off what they thought might lead them to bad news – suspecting or fearing that they were indeed terminally ill. I can well understand these hesitators who self-torture themselves with fear of what could happen when they do turn up. These were maybe the ones postponing because of their dread not only of treatment required but preferring not to know how poorly they were.

Lose the fear. That's your new mantra. Don't be a scaredy cat.

At the very start I knew I had to beat my aversion to white coats, doctors, nurses and hospital buildings, medical equipment, needles, scalpels and surgeries. Immediately in my head I began the process.

I focused on the person I was dealing with at appointments, be it a man or a woman. The uniform they were wearing was to become incidental. The person treating me had gone into the caring profession, and undergone substantial training and become a doctor, a radiologist a nurse, all expert in their field to help me and others through concerning times of poor health like my own.

The tools they used, the needles and scalpels, were not what I used to perceive them as – instruments of torture, they were tools for good, tools of their trade.

From the start I got used to having my blood taken. You'd better get used to giving blood because the health service sucks it out of its patients to check your state of health but do so with the appetite of a vampire cult.

Of course, in an emergency – sometimes in a lifesaving situation – they pump blood into us.

Blood is taken and given all the time. Our blood tells doctors such a lot about our ailments. The queues to give blood in the hospital are some of the longest you will join. And blood is still being taken from me now as an outpatient. I've had it taken dozens and dozens of times by so many nurses and I can report that most of them scored 9 out of 10 for compassion. "You'll just feel a scratch," they tell you and that in the main is exactly all you put up with. I had many a cannula on my arm so they could inject me with the substances that they put inside of you for instance when undergoing the MRI or CT scans.

The diagnosis of bowel cancer was confirmed after a second colonoscopy this time under a general anaesthetic. The first colonoscopy, although it didn't work for me under a sedative, as the discomfort was too great, had given me the diagnosis of bowel cancer.

I must have been moaning during the procedure. I didn't recall complaining of discomfort at any time. This 'discomfort' was written on my report. I can't recall either though having had any pleasant or unpleasant dreams.

My next colonoscopy examination was under general anaesthetic. What happens during a general? You remember nothing. You are out like a light, as if you have been floored by a well delivered hook from world title fighter Tyson Fury, but without feeling the pain of a punch like his. The period you are unconscious seems to have been all of five seconds before you are awake again. Then whatever procedure you were undergoing is over.

So why worry yourself sick beforehand. Just go and have it done. In a blink it is over, especially under a general anaesthetic.

It was a fortnight prior to Christmas day 2022 that I was diagnosed with cancer and from then on it felt as if I'd been enlisted in well drilled army. Information about what to do and not to do was never lacking. It is sent by letter or sometimes in texts or by e-mail to your home address and booklets arrived, explaining how to get support of any kind if you need it. It was, as I say, as if I had signed up for the military.

I must admit I stockpiled most of this information to read if I felt I needed to read it. Reading the whole lot would have been like picking up The Bible or War and Peace. Don't suffer information overload and probably best not to Google to discover how other patients handled being diagnosed and treated with your condition. You can easily be led astray by misinformation out there especially from pessimists or conspiracy theorists on the superhighway.

Though usually in my life I would describe myself as a devil's advocate practitioner, a humourist, and a sometimes rebel. I knew at this point of my life I had to get serious. I would not slow the process or time waste by being an awkward customer. The people I was consulting with were experts in their field. I would ask only needful questions and follow instructions to the letter. The NHS too, as you are all aware, is a very busy service and queues are also there to remind you of that. Remember on entering you are just one of tens of thousands going through similar treatment although you may think of yourself as the only one and maybe even the priority.

Fitting in and not wasting medical staff time helps others.

I had undertaken the MRI and CT scans to identify if the cancer had spread to other parts of my body. In other words, what Grade was it? Grade 4 or 5 is not good. Initially I scored a two, quite promising. Later doctors discovered it was more complicated.

From my test results they couldn't quite see from the scans or decide what to do until the operation itself revealed just what was going on inside of me.

The surgeon prepped to do surgery at Stepping Hill Hospital Stockport eventually told me that having seen the scans the care team treating me had decided that it would probably need two surgeons with expertise at the better equipped Christie Hospital, in Manchester. The bowel tumour on the scans seemed to be burrowing through the wall of the prostate. It wasn't conclusive one way or the other.

The Christie is the hospital attached to the Paterson Institute, the scientific arm for cancer research where I used to visit during my days with Cancer Research UK to interview scientists based there from all over the world who were funded by the charity to carry out their work. I found myself back on home ground.

It was a little unnerving to change consultants halfway through, but what is, is and you must go with it. Move on.

I went to The Christie and at an initial meeting with two doctors I was read the terms of a contract that I was expected to sign accepting the treatment they had outlined for me. It was a very long contract. I had been presented with similar contracts by salespeople in my dim past when purchasing furniture on hire purchase.

The two female doctors present wanted to make sure I understood the negative aspects of my treatment, and they were there to explain any detail, anything in fact I couldn't understand. There was a lot to take in. So much information can seem overwhelming. Sometimes you come out of a meeting like this and only then think of all the questions that perhaps you would have liked to have asked or should have. Write these down and ask away on your next visit. They'll give you the answers and put your mind at rest if need be.

There are a lot of consultations prior to treatment. You may even be appointed a liaison nurse to be your main point of contact at the hospital. It's better, if possible, when you attend appointments to have someone with you. Four ears are better than two.

I've been told by others facing interviews that a patient can retain the good bits of what he hears and conveniently forgets the bad bits. You'll need someone to remind you, gently, of the less positive aspects they hear of your medical prospects.

However, consider this. Whenever we're prescribed a pill, most of us swallow it on trust believing doctor knows best and that is what you must get used to doing. Who reads the small print on the notes inside drug packaging anyway? Dare we read them? Everything comes with a warning of some sort the days.

Most of these warnings are as applicable or meritorious as someone pointing out that you might get knocked down by a bus coming out of the hospital.

After being told of the negative effects of treatment and especially radiotherapy I was asked to sign the contract.

This was the moment I referred to earlier when I was told the truth about my cancer.

"What happens if I don't sign the contract?" I asked.

"The cancer will kill you," one of the doctor's replied.

I signed on that line quickly. "Let's get it done."

Though I had undergone MRI and CT scans at Stockport now they wanted to repeat them once more at Christie. They also wanted to do further exploration under a general anaesthetic to study what the tumour was up to inside of me before they did the surgery.

As scans were inconclusive, my new consultant told me at a pre op meeting: "You are going to have to write me a blank cheque and I will deal accordingly with what I find." This was rather like a shotgun wedding.

They were to find quite a lot…

What they had decided to do initially at Stockport was to zap the beast with a combination of chemotherapy and radiotherapy and then remove it with surgery. I was in for the full whammy. The radiotherapy was to be five weeks of five days every week at the Christie Hospital in Manchester, which is one of the UK's and Europe's leading cancer hospitals.

The Christie is a fine modern place, nothing like the crumbling, Dickensian hospitals I managed to avoid for so long and that I remembered well from my stay, again as a child in an isolation unit to recover from chicken pox complications – and at yet another hospital to have my tonsils removed. Was there any wonder I had white coat syndrome since childhood.

After the marathon radiotherapy and chemotherapy treatment I was informed they had done a good job on shrinking the tumour, but it still needed to be operated on to be removed.

I received instructions to my home address of what I would need to take with me for an approximate 10 day stay at Christie hospital when I would have the operation and an overnight stay in critical care after surgery.

Now what I always appreciated throughout treatment was when there was the relief of a week or two or even just days between appointments, the joy of having a weekend free before further bouts of radiotherapy for instance was bliss. In my mind, that time was to be enjoyed and not a time for worry. But it's difficult not to countdown the days and become preoccupied with negative thoughts and to be more nervous as hospital appointment time draws ever closer.

Think ahead instead. Fill your head with good stuff. Why not do some future planning? Plan where to go and what to do when treatment is complete. Time will fly by. Give yourself goals. Go for it.

What I began to appreciate is how time between appointments really does fly ever so quickly. No sooner is one appointment ticked off than the countdown to the next begins. This was a comfort.

All things pass and they pass particularly fast when you're on a hospital conveyer belt. Using this knowledge my surgery would be over in no time. And do you know what? It was and it will be for you too.

Treatment from beginning to its end was, I deemed it, going to be a brief interlude in my life. I just had to turn up. I was not going to be in a hospital bed for any longer than my presence was urgently required because the hospital is so short of beds for the next patients, they are queuing to climb into them. Trust me your consultant or the doctors will want to get you out of that bed and home as sharpish as possible even if you do happen to be a big hit with the nurses and doctors because you don't grumble and you're nice and joke along with them.

This speed of turnover of patients you will witness, and you will be involved in after you've had major surgery. It seems before you've blinked an eye or moved one little finger on your first feeble step to recovery the physiotherapy team are there at your bedside in their distinctive uniforms wanting you to get out of your bed and to sit you up in a chair.

This they assure you is for the good of your health. You certainly don't feel that way as you are disorientated and attached to tubes that are feeding you and you are probably feeling as I was dizzy and as feeble as a new-born kitten.

All you want to do is to get back into bed and sleep, but you can't even move from the chair back into the bed without the physio's assistance. You can't do a thing for yourself apart from breathe, and that may be a struggle. You are dependent.

In the soonest time possible time this physio team will want to have you walking. First to the bathroom, perhaps with a helping arm. Even the tiniest steps are celebrated with as much gusto as do men or women applauded for conquering the peak of a monster mountain.

After you have mastered walking again, the physios unveil to you their acid test which is your personal mountain to climb – they want to watch you cope with the hospital stairs. Climb a couple of flights of these and you've made it. Climb those and you are a man or a woman my friend and yours is the earth and everything in it. Wasn't that quoting the poet Kipling?

After I had done my stairs trial I was signed off as being mobile, but they still insist you keep on walking everywhere and do it any opportunity you get every day you are on the ward. You must make it a habit. They want that bed of yours...

Now having come out of that long tunnel of treatment myself and having first hated then appreciated that physiotherapy team,

I say to all scaredy cats, worry is your chief enemy and to curtail worrying beforehand you must find ways to occupy your mind and body with either exercise or hobbies, sewing, knitting, books and music and good company.

Whatever it takes for you to stay upbeat – do it! Remember this treatment is going to be good for you. Do it the right way without worrying unnecessarily and its over in a flash.

Here's a further hint though. You can have bags and bags of sympathy from family and friends if you want it, you know you can. You just let everyone who knows you know, in the greatest detail what you are going through. You could share your grimaces and tears after diagnosis. But think of it this way. If everyone knows about your illness, then everyone is going to ask you how you are feeling or coping each time they see or speak to you.

They'll feel it necessary each time you meet them to ask you how you are. Do you want to be spoken to as a sick person by everyone you know? I found it easier to tell just a few people and explain to them that I didn't want a fuss.

That way it's taking control.

Select a close circle to tell and hopefully they will be supportive when you do need moral support or practical help, but you may need less support than you think if you're not obsessing about it and instead getting on with other things.

I'd meet people in the town where I live who knew me well enough, but who I'd deliberately left in the dark about my circumstances.

"How are you?" they'd ask.

"Great," I'd reply.

"You look good," they'd say.

That's good, I'd think. They wouldn't have said that had they known what was wrong with me.

My plan 'A' worked. Only tell people you are ill on a need-to-know basis.

Hundreds of thousands of patients have been through the treatments that you are about to go through. Medical staff carrying out these procedures could probably manage them in their sleep (well not quite). Just don't worry. Listen and collect in your memory the positive vibes you are given along the way and if you do listen, you'll discover there are many positive things to take on board.

Listen for the positive vibes.

These people looking after you give out positive vibes because they want you to cope and be upbeat and they do care about your welfare.

Another hint I was given was when you go to hospital is leave yourself at the door and collect yourself when you leave.

Throughout my career I had been a journalist questioning everything. Now my philosophy for dealing with this was different. Less questions and more listening and action on my part was required. Turn up. I was putting my faith in the experts. I was going to be I hoped the model patient! I felt I managed it.

More hints for you scaredy cats later, but first…

CHAPTER THREE

PREDICTING 9/11... AND MY OWN DEMISE

I had been diagnosed with cancer and that just happened to correspond with me also being informed I was going to have a book I had written, published – I had titled my book long before I knew I had cancer 'Reincarnation for Beginners'.

Now I had been told face to face by a doctor: "The cancer will kill you unless you have the tumour removed."

Was the title of my book prophetic? Had I foreseen my departure from this life and was I to be re-incarnated – and for the very first time? More interestingly, as what or who would I return?

The doctor had given me my choice. Not a great one, in fact he left me with no choice at all really. It was either 25 sessions of radiotherapy over five weeks along with doses of chemotherapy and then the removal of the tumour under general anaesthetic – or death.

Did I want to live or die?

Soon enough I'd signed up for the operation.

Now while I was waiting for my major op and knowing I was going to have to keep myself from worrying unnecessarily, I went otherworldly busy by starting to write my next story, a

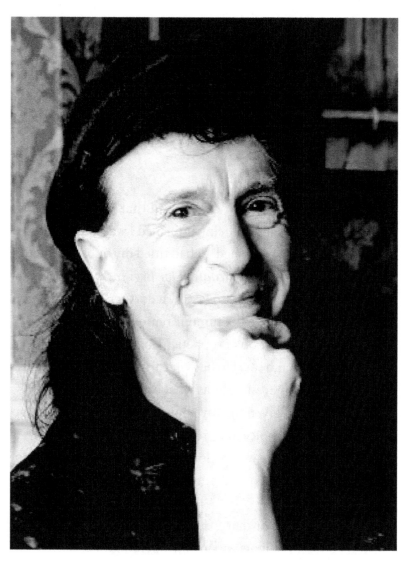

Alan Charnley as author Marmaduke Jinks.

follow up to the one just accepted by the publisher. To cheer me up this would be comic and have nothing to do with death or re-incarnation. I began to lose myself in my imagination and creativity.

This was a great distraction.

Throughout my life I have always been a professional writer and when I wasn't working in journalism or public relations for cancer charities, I was writing fiction or song writing. I have written plays and musicals, but now I was wondering even at this early stage of my cancer if it was mere coincidence or whether I had bizarrely predicted my own demise in '*Reincarnation for Beginners*'.

It wasn't a good title to go out on, but then again it might have been the best!?...

In fact, that book I had written, which will come out under my author's name of Marmaduke Jinks, was far from fatalistic or glum. It was comic and quirky. Essentially it was about characters trying to understand or come to terms with who they were and or finding happiness or belief in the fact they believed themselves to be someone else or very similar to someone else who had lived before.

It was okay in my book for believers in *Muff's Theory*, as I called it, if someone believed they were Napoleon reincarnated. They weren't barmy if they kept within the bounds of the law and didn't raise an army to kill a rival person who contrastingly believed himself to be the reincarnation of Wellington.

But no, I didn't start believing that I'd return to earth after my own death from cancer as Elvis Presley or Buddy Holly.

This book title 'coincidence' of mine was no great surprise as similar things had occurred before. Yes, I had written 'clairvoyantly' before, but especially on one occasion.

Go on, ask me about the time I wrote a comedy book called 'Cosmic Lives' about three air stewardesses who prevented a plane on a suicide mission from being crashed into the Statue of Liberty!

In my plot a small army, knowing it was too under resourced and under manned to go to war with a Goliath state like the United States chose instead to make a strategic strike on a proposed suicide mission to the iconic heart of a US city.

My story was written before 9/11. It was completed and ready for send-off to a list of publishers just days before 9/11.

My chirpy story ended well and happily enough – but 9/11 didn't. It was a day of tragedy and horror.

My 100,000-word manuscript was about to be dispatched when two suicide mission planes unbelievably struck the Twin Towers in Manhattan.

My comedy book from then on could only have been read as having been written in poor or cruel taste and written too after 9/11 happened and not before. Nobody could have foreseen 9/11 happening, could they? Certainly, American national defences weren't prepared for it.

But I had written my story before the real true-life event occurred, my wife Gillian knows it and the dates on the copy prove it. I had written the 'unbelievable' from my imagination and now it had occurred in real life just a few miles from the Statue of Liberty, my book's plane suicide mission target.

I wasn't the first to do this.

An author did the same in the dim and distant past when he wrote about the fictional Titan passenger ship sinking 20 years before the actual Titanic sank killing more than a thousand passengers and crew.

It took me several years to fulfil an ambition to write a novel and complete 'Cosmic Lives' then on 9/11 it had to be binned.

I was working for Cancer Research Campaign at Salford Quays Manchester when 9/11 occurred and my wife Gillian called me at the charity's office.

"Have you got the television on," she asked.

I looked up from my computer. I hadn't been watching it, but I noticed a crowd of our charity workers had gathered around a TV set in the office and were glued to the screen.

"Your story has come true – the script that we are about to send out as fictional comedy has happened," Gillian continued.

"What do you mean?" I asked, still in the dark.

"Cosmic Lives. Your plane was going to crash in a suicide mission into the Statue of Liberty. It's only gone and happened in real life just a few miles away. A plane has gone crashing into one of the Twin Towers in Manhattan."

Everyone now knows that second suicide mission plane followed, of course, hitting the second tower.

"We can't send the book out now. The FBI will want to be questioning you wondering if you planned or knew about the real thing," Gillian said.

She was serious. She was right. In this instance truth was certainly stranger than fiction.

Incidentally, I am now living next to a church that happens to be identical to the one I used to draw and paint all the time from my imagination when I was attending a South Yorkshire primary school.

I lived miles away from this church in Derbyshire and had never seen it as a child. I always painted covered in snow. Does this have a meaning now; I wonder?

CHAPTER FOUR

MEETING INSPIRATIONAL CANCER PATIENTS

Who'd have thought that when I became a journalist, I would end up writing and working for cancer charities, I certainly never did, and I hadn't sought employment with them either just because my dad had died from cancer, but who knows if the work I did for the charities paid dividends for me and gave me courage I didn't know I had when cancer did come my way.

Some of the fortitude I have shown during my own treatment that surprised even me may have resulted because I interviewed brave and inspirational people along the way who live long in my memory. Here are the stories of just two of them.

They may inspire you too.

One morning, working for Cancer Research Campaign at their Salford Quays office I received a telephone call from someone informing me about a young girl called Natalie who lived in Stockport. She loved football and playing the game and was 13.

But cancer had struck the youngster and it led to the amputation of one of her legs.

It got me thinking. Did her involvement in football, the game she loved necessarily need to end now?

I was doing a spot of what they call blue-sky thinking. Blue sky thinking was all the rage then. Thinking outside the box. Most employees though used blue sky thinking as an excuse to take a snooze.

What about Natalie going into football management, I thought?

Okay that idea was way before its time, but Natalie had done very well for herself getting game time in her day because women's or girls' football was not as popular or promoted as it is today. There were fewer opportunities then.

But I didn't hesitate in getting in touch with the football club just across from my office at nearby Old Trafford. I asked could I speak to Sir Alex Ferguson? "What! You wanted to speak to him? A legend?" Mm, of course not everyone could get access to speak to that giant of a football manager, considered one of the best of all time. I took my place in a queue to speak to an underling at the club instead.

I told her: "I'm from Cancer Research Campaign and I have a girl who is football mad and as she's had to have her leg amputated because of cancer, she's considering football management. There's surely no finer person in this country or perhaps in the world is there to give her a little bit of advice in that department but Sir Alex? Could you ask him if he'll give her a few tips in person?"

"I will ask him," she replied.

If the man had a heart, which I was sure he had that would be enough for him to get back to me.

It was the following day I got a call from Manchester United with a message from Sir Alex: "Bring Natalie in."

I broke the news to Natalie and was that girl excited! She was so thrilled she might have been celebrating scoring the winning goal in the cup final at Wembley.

The date was fixed, and she was invited to attend the Manchester United training ground where she met the players and was shown around and was gifted a football kit and a team autographed ball by Sir Alex himself who was generous with his time and kindliness itself to Natalie and her accompanying family. I was full of admiration for the man.

Sometimes notorious for his dealings with the media, Sir Alex was then not speaking to the press, he made an exception for our cancer charity on that day, and we got great coverage for Natalie's story both locally and nationally. Natalie was as pleased as punch.

It was maybe 12 months or more later that I visited a children's cancer hospital ward when a slim emaciated girl who had lost her hair, obviously because of chemotherapy approached me.

"Do you remember me?" she asked me.

I'm afraid I didn't because she had lost so much weight and had changed so much. I didn't let on I didn't recognize her. "Of course." I replied.

"Of course, I do. How are you?"

She told me how she was very poorly. Cancer had returned with a vengeance.

I had been buying time as I talked to her. I was hoping my memory would click into gear. Who was this delightful girl?

It only registered after I had left the ward and was heading home in the car after bidding her goodbye.

It was Natalie. She died shortly after, but what a brave, lovely and delightful girl she was.

And how sorry I was that I couldn't have talked football with her that day.

Then there was another cancer victim.

One morning, while working for Cancer Research UK, I picked up an early morning e-mail which started: "Please help me I am dying." It was from Susan Price from Manchester who had been given six months to live and was being denied a new drug that might have extended her life only because of where she lived.

The most wonderful thing about being a journalist was always having the clout to help people who had no-one else to help them. Doing this led to the best and most memorable days spent in my profession – and I'm thankful these days occurred quite often. They do if you are a watchful journalist and keep an eye out for these stories. In the profession they call it having a good news sense. The joy to me was the privilege of taking the side of an underdog who had a genuine cause or complaint against powers that be who were being neglectful in their duty. Shaming them in the newspaper in fact. Yes, it was satisfying using journalism to help others but also at the same time it gave me great stories. It was win-win.

I remember my early days in journalism on the 100,000 a day circulation Sheffield Star and I was one of a team of three reporters working on a consumer problems page.

We had clout in those days. I got people new washing machines, cars, TV's, holidays, you name it – and I did it daily when consumers complained to us about the shoddy goods they had been sold or bad deals they had fallen foul of.

When Susan Price sent her email, I wasted no time and immediately spoke to her on the phone and inspired by her I wrote a story which I then sent out to the regional and national press who followed it up and used it bigtime.

Susan could have bought the drug she needed privately but how could she or other women in the same boat afford it. It was £800 for the first treatment and thereafter £400 a week for as long as she lived. Herceptin was out there and was shown to have increased the life span of women cancer patients – but some got it, but others didn't, dependent on where they lived. It was a post code lottery.

Susan, with her life ebbing away wanted to campaign to show the injustice of this post code lottery unfair drug availability. She would be the arrowhead of this unfair injustice.

Once the media got hold of my story, other women in Manchester and nationally came forward to tell of their disappointment at not being allowed Herceptin and how the decision was going to shorten their precious lives.

One result of the ensuing publicity drive was that health chiefs in Manchester made Herceptin available to women in the city who couldn't previously access or afford it.

Susan sadly died but was responsible for helping fellow breast cancer sufferers by going public with her story. A determined and brave woman she successfully fought an injustice.

I was being appraised by my boss Joanna Lavelle on the day the media went mad with the story to tell Susan's heartbreak story. I was excusing myself throughout the interview with Joanna as the phone never stopped ringing as I fielded calls from media all over the UK.

The media is an important and vital tool to achieving fairness and much more locally and in world affairs. Long may it remain free and accurate in unsettling times.

CHAPTER FIVE

WAS MY CANCER CAUSED BY A BOMB DROPPED ON JAPAN?

My unusual link with cancer, and the possibility that there is or was a hereditary reason that I developed the disease is strange but true and dates all the way back to the Americans dropping the Atom bomb on the fishing port of Nagasaki in 1945.

That bomb was called The Fat Man and it was the dad I never knew who developed cancer after he went to serve with his army regiment in that devastated city in Japan.

What causes our cancer tumours anyway or why do we get them? What led to mine? They will always ask you at the hospital if there is cancer in your family to determine if it could be hereditary.

I told doctors my dad had been riddled with it after serving in Japan. My mother had breast cancer too.

As a child growing up, my mother used to fear there was a ticking time bomb inside of me, but I wasn't aware of this family history until I was an adult. My mother kept it from me. My father died from his cancer when I was just a baby, weeks old.

His was caused by radiation poisoning from working in an area where the bomb had fallen.

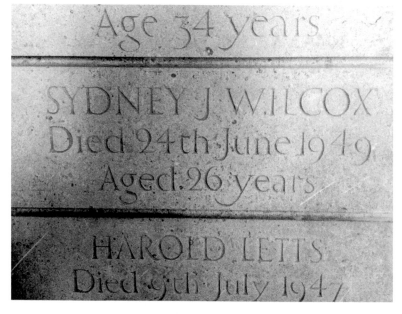

Forgotten soldier: Sydney Wilcox memorial stone in Birmingham.

I was born just weeks before my dad Sydney Joseph Wilcox died, aged 26, in a Birmingham hospital following his return from Japan. I'd be fortunate not to have caught cancer if it is hereditary.

When I was conceived, he was riddled with cancer, but because the atomic bomb and radiation poisoning was new, he wouldn't have known he was a dying man.

When they operated on my tumour, I was hoping they would discover it bore a label saying Made in Japan to prove my case conclusively.

But let's go back to 1945, four years before I was born.

Sydney Joseph Wilcox, who was with the Royal Engineers, was on a boat to a secret destination. He had hurriedly married my mother. He had been told his regiment were about to be posted abroad but that it was top secret. Soldiers were to be kept in the dark that it was Japan.

Syd hadn't a clue what to tell Judy when she asked him about his destination. But powers that be had designated that he and his fellow soldiers be sent to Hiroshima or Nagasaki. The troops mission was to clean up, repair infrastructure, construct bridges literally, as well as build bridges by offering the hand of friendship to the traumatized Japanese people still alive in these devastated cities after the dropping by the Americans of their two atom bombs.

Nagasaki where my father was dispatched was a capital for shipbuilding and a fishing port. That atom bomb, the second ever dropped by a specially adapted B-29 bomber called 'Bock's Car', took off from Tinian Island under the command of Maj. Charles W. Sweeney. The bomb was dropped at 11:02 a.m., 1,650 feet above the city.

The explosion unleashed the equivalent force of 22,000 tons of TNT. Surrounding hills did a better job of containing the destructive force, but the human toll in the city itself was catastrophic. Burned and battered corpses littered the rubble of the destroyed Japanese cities. Some 90,000 corpses in the case of Hiroshima, with a further 75,000 in Nagasaki. Exact figures are impossible, the blast having obliterated bodies and destroyed records. Men, women and children lay burned and dead.

A US Nagasaki army veteran later testified. "You had to be there to understand what it did. We did not drop those two bombs on military installations. We dropped them on women and children… I think that is something America is going to have to live with for eternity."

While this second bomb was bringing terror and death to the streets of Nagasaki, my mother to be, Gladys Judith Dunham was serving in the women's ATS corps. My father to be she had met in a workshop where he repaired vehicles while soldiering with the Royal Engineers. She admits to lingering in that workshop to be around him and sometimes was the butt of sexist and suggestive remarks from some of the men. Syd told them to button their lips in a lady's presence, indicating he was no shrinking violet and a gentleman.

My mother said she had dropped enough hints to Syd that she fancied him: "It took him ages to ask me out," she complained to me later.

Syd played piano and led a concert party playing for troops at their own camp and others. Syd had taken piano lessons while young and could play classical pieces. Now for fellow soldiers unused to classical music he played the pop songs of his day.

I was to discover much later Gladys – she always used the name Judy – and Sydney Joseph Wilcox's concert act in the army was singing as Flanagan and Allen, popular artistes of the time. Away from Flanagan & Allen, who were the Morecambe and Wise of their time, the pair's 'special' sentimental love song shared together was a hit record of the time '*Love Letters in The Sand*'.

Romance blossomed between the two and then young soldier boy Syd, 23, from Wednesbury, Staffs, heard about his posting.

Judy told me on Facebook: "Syd begged me to marry him before he went. It was all very hush hush where he was going to be posted."

The couple did marry and honeymooned in Blackpool. Exactly where I honeymooned just over 20 years later, but I wasn't aware of that coincidence because my mother had shut the door on her past and locked it when Syd died.

Weeks later fate decided that Sydney Joseph Wilcox was one of the 2,000 expeditionary force sent from Britain to Japan.

What about Syd's cancer? Was it an inevitable prelude to my own? Did it increase the odds of myself or his grandchildren inheriting the disease?

According to historical reports, which are sketchy, British servicemen underwent regular checks for radiation poisoning, carried out by US Army medics, while they were stationed in Japan.

The Allies were instructed not to drink the local water but to use their own supply. My mother told some she knew that on his return Syd had told her he had drank the water.

He must have seen a lot of things in a short space of time that I suppose no-one should see in their lifetime.

After the dead had been buried and the wounded had been sent to the few medical facilities available, the task of surveying and clearing the vast fields of rubble and debris began. This process took the better part of two years to complete. First, the rubble was cleared from the major streets, allowing trucks and heavy equipment better access to the site. By March of 1946, the main roads have been cleared of debris, and many of the ruined buildings have been demolished and cleared away. This being done, it was possible to start restoring the infrastructure necessary to rebuild the city, the water and sewage lines, electrical lines and food distribution.

It was in Nagasaki that Sydney contracted cancer. Just three years later and now getting treatment at the Queen Elizabeth Hospital, Birmingham his body was ravaged by the disease. At 26 he was dying from radiation poisoning.

Just weeks before he died, I was born and according to my mother he was only well enough to hold me in his arms just the once. She later changed that story to Syd never having had the chance to hold me at all because he was too weak. As a child I was never sure what to believe because my mother covered up true facts until late in life.

Of course, the atomic bomb was a new weapon and its gruesome effects had not yet been realized.

The hundreds upon hundreds of soldiers in Birmingham alone who crowded the hospital wards were not accepted as victims of cancer or disease due to their army service in Japan. They were not compensated. Nobody was taking responsibility for this disaster for mankind apart from the originator of the atom bomb Robert Oppenheimer known as the 'father of the atomic bomb'. He had watched the first test of that bomb from hell in a vast desert in Mexico. According to reports it created a mushroom cloud climbing 40,000 feet.

Oppenheimer that day recited a piece of Hindu scripture: "Now I am become death, the destroyer of worlds."

In recent times Putin in Russia held the world to ransom with nuclear threat, those words Oppenheimer used still ring true and the fear for humanity is the worst is always yet to come. New generations cannot even imagine the scale or horror of current nuclear weapons. If used, they would be even far more horrific and potent than those used in Japan.

If Japan had surrendered after the dropping of the bomb on Hiroshima, then the American's said they would never have dropped the second bomb on Nagasaki, but they did and they did it only three days later. By doing so they changed hundreds of thousands of lives by their action including my own.

In the USA and Japan since the dropping of those first atomic bombs there has been more research on men who have been exposed to nuclear radiation, especially in Japan. It has been established that it might not just be the children of radiation victims but the grandchildren who in some cases inherit deformities from genetic impact.

Of my children from my first marriage to Anne – she and I married straight out of school as teenagers – my daughter was born with an extra kidney and went on to receive cancer treatment, my eldest son was born with extra teeth and recently had a pre-cancerous polyp removed from his bowel, and my younger son suffers with serious eye, and ear and spine problems while my youngest daughter from my second marriage also has spine and kidney issues – yet none of these conditions in my children

53

can be checked or linked to what happened to my father. But they may be linked, as now might my own cancer.

When I had the first three children during my first marriage, I was unaware of my dad's cancer and the radiation link. Had I been aware of this link would I have taken a decision as an adult not to risk having children? Who knows? But being an impetuous youth maybe I wouldn't have, and they are great kids who enjoy their own lives. But should the choice have been mine alone? Shouldn't my wife Anne have been informed of my progeny and the risk? My mother had chosen to keep this a secret from me and my wife, so the subject was never up for discussion. Secrecy was my mum's way of dealing with difficult issues.

Author Greg Mitchell is one of the few who has tackled this silent topic of the Japanese bomb drops, the truth of which many soldier took to their graves – that they died from cancers caused by the atomic bomb.

Mitchell's book is '*Atomic Cover Up: Hiroshima & Nagasaki – The Greatest Movie Never Made*'.

He points out that every major story in the history of mankind has been made into a film – so why hasn't the American attack on Japan with atomic bombs reached the silver screen. Is it because the victor writes the history?

The American film industry has peddled '*Pearl Harbour*' and '*Tora, Tora, Tora*' from the US standpoint, celebrating revenge and victory. What about the story told from on the ground in Hiroshima and Nagasaki and from the standpoint of innocent Japanese survivors, the women and children and those allied soldiers who unknowingly were sacrificing their lives in the post-bomb clean-up but are now a forgotten generation ignored and not celebrated in the history books – like my dad.

After the atomic bombs dropped there were reports of the people of Hiroshima and Nagasaki being afflicted by a deadly plague, but this was reported by the Americans as Japanese propaganda.

An Australia journalist Wilfred Burchett was the first to file a story for the *Daily Express* about the 'atomic plague'.

However, US radiologists and physicists said it was safe for allied soldiers to go there because no poisonous gases had been detected and vegetation was growing.

Allied troops were not told to take precautions. They cleared bodies without protective clothing and some even slept on poisoned ground.

US soldiers quoted in Greg Mitchell's book said.

"We walked into Nagasaki unprepared… Really, we were ignorant about what the hell the bomb was."

Another vet said: "Hell, we drank the water, we breathed the air, and we lived in the rubble. We did our duty."

A marine named Sam Scione, who had survived battles on Guadalcanal, Tarawa and Okinawa, now arrived in Nagasaki, sleeping first in a burned-out factory, then a schoolhouse. "We never learned anything about radiation or the effects it might have on us," he later said. "We went to ground zero many times and were never instructed not to go there." A year later, on his return to the United States, his hair began to fall out and his body was covered in sores. He suffered a string of ailments but never was awarded service-related disability status.

The occupying force in Nagasaki grew to more than 27,000.

The horrors of Hiroshima and Nagasaki are not completely forgotten but were they to have had the highly merited and continued media exposure of say the concentration camps in World War Two and the Holocaust, there might be more focus now to avoid nuclear conflict in the future at all costs and less threats made by careless tongued, war-mongering politicians threatening that nuclear weapons could be used if certain lines are crossed. Conventional war is bad enough, but nuclear war's effect on humanity would be indescribably horrific.

The story of what happened to the tens of thousands of innocent victims walking the streets of those Japanese cities when the bombs dropped should be evermore more widely circulated. The accounts of what the allied troops saw when they got there and what they experienced afterwards in terms of illnesses including cancer should too have been told. Instead, it was brushed under the carpet.

Sometimes we stand too close to the threshold of potential nuclear disaster. Too perilously close to the edge!

It was suggested in the day that Nagasaki should have been preserved exactly as it was after the bomb had hit. Future peace conferences could then be held there, it was suggested, in the ashy, desolated, sea of rubble to make politicians fearful of repeating nuclear attacks. They didn't go ahead with that because they said politicians might feel 'uncomfortable' in such a setting. How sensitive of them!

Despite the efforts of a Committee for US Veterans of Hiroshima and Nagasaki to win disability and compensation their claims were denied. British troops from that time have also been denied.

They even had a book published in 1982 called '*Killing Their Own*'. US radiation victims were consistently ignored and denied at every turn by the very institutions responsible for causing their problems, they claimed.

In summary the dropping of that atomic bomb is the reason I never met my father. He was destroyed by a cancer caused by radiation poisoning. It was a new bomb so when the casualties came back to the UK surgeons experimented medically upon soldiers like my father.

My mother told me in a letter late in life that she told the hospital not to medically experiment on Syd. He has suffered enough, she told them.

They went ahead after Syd's dad gave permission.

My father was cut apart and my mother saw him sewed back together in the coffin.

Am I angry? At an injustice, yes!

Is there any remembrance or thanks to my father for sacrificing his life to help the victims and people of Japan? Nope.

Is there any recognition of what poverty, struggle and strife was experienced by families of those who lost husbands and parents? No there wasn't. Those politically responsible for colluding in this neglect should have hung their heads in shame.

There is little enough written about these forgotten heroes of war, but you can wise up by reading this…

Greg Mitchell's book and e-book is Atomic Cover-up: Two U.S. Soldiers, Hiroshima & Nagasaki and The Greatest Movie Never Told.

CHAPTER SIX

MUM DECIDED TO KILL US BOTH

Left alone with a baby after my father's death from cancer caused by the radiation poisoning my mother Judy was depressed. She decided she had taken enough of what life had to offer her and decided to kill us both.

My mother was understandably depressed after Sydney's horrible and traumatic death. He was the first real love of her life.

One night she had prepared herself mentally for our demise. Her plan was to close all the windows and doors and seal ventilation points in the kitchen and to then switch on the gas oven which would see us both off.

Before she went ahead with it however, she took a walk in the night air outside walking me along the street in a pram. When she returned to the house, she looked at me and thankfully couldn't bring herself to do it. She says I saved her that night. Such is the hand of fate.

That story having been shared with me as a child or when I was old enough to hear it, would have forged a bond between my mother and I… but she never told me until too late in the day.

My father dying from cancer had a profound effect on my mother who was then only in her early 20's herself when it happened. Syd's loss shaped her. The loss of a loved one shapes anyone. But the love and loss of Syd became her secret and hers alone from then on. She decided it was best kept that way even when she remarried shortly afterwards. Of course, Terry would have known about Syd because I was there as the living proof, but I wonder how much else she kept from Terry because he was a jealous man, as most men can be.

However, keeping the secret of Syd's life and death and how she suppressed emotions from then on in her life, I maintain sowed the seed for our eventual estrangement that lasted 50 plus years.

Yes, you heard that right. 50 years!

It nearly lasted an entire lifetime and if someone had suggested at any stage that we might have one day called a truce I would have laughed or cried or explained why I thought we had left it far too late.

But we made it back together by messaging on Facebook.

You see, when aged 91 my mother sought me out on Facebook. I was 66 and we began a journey to make sense of the years we spent apart. Around eighty thousand words later we did bury the hatchet, but more of that later.

Music as you will now know brought Syd and Judy together.

In the early 1970's when I was married with three young children after buying a new home, I had bought myself an old piano from a local church. I was then around 23 years old – the age my mum had lost Syd, but I didn't know that. I had no clue of my family history!

My mother visited me at the house shortly after my piano's installation. I had already painted it white. I was sat there teaching myself how to play when she arrived. I was self-taught on the piano and worked out chord shapes to back any new songs I was writing. I always had song ideas buzzing inside my head like bees in a hive. Out of the blue my mother informed me: "Your dad used to play the piano."

Wow. That came like a bolt out of the blue.

That was the first I knew of it. AND we never talked about HIM.

You see my whole life since Syd's death had been lived in the dark my mother keeping the tightest lid on my past, on Syd's existence, her past life and on her own emotions.

But what a fascinating and valuable piece information I had just heard! A piece of a jigsaw. A building brick in knowing who my father was. I had inherited a musical gene from the dad I never met and who I knew next to nothing about. What a revelation when I was told!

But why wasn't I told sooner?

A few years earlier, on a whim, I had named my baby son and middle child Joseph not knowing that it just happened to be Syd's middle name too. The name 'Joseph' came to me as I walking to the register office because my wife Anne and I had decided upon Terry as one name because both 'grandads' bore that name.

I only found out that Syd bore the name Joseph very late in life too when I saw my own original birth certificate which I hadn't known existed. That original bore my own name which wasn't

Alan Philip Charnley as is now, but Alan Sydney Wilcox and Syd's middle name was there for me to see too, Joseph.

That original birth certificate I hadn't known had existed. I hadn't had sight of it either because it had been superseded by my adoption birth certificate and that later version is what I was sent when I required a replacement.

That Sydney's middle name was Joseph and my mother had never told me – or told my son Joe that he bore the same name as his late grandad I regarded as strange to say the least. I think that my choice of Joe's name must have been Syd giving me a gentle nudge from somewhere out in the cosmos. He wasn't going to remain forgotten. My mother however was making sure that he was.

Mother gave me no further nuggets of information during further visits to my house visiting her grandchildren, but I wished she had revealed to me sooner that my dad played piano more especially since my stepfather Terry had already told me when I was a boy that he didn't like music, a fact I found unbelievable so that's probably why I remembered the conversation we had so well. No-one else on earth since has told me since that they don't like music. I thought everybody must at least like some kind of music even if they aren't in love with it as I was. I adored music.

Therefore, I deduced, my gift of music hadn't come to me as a direct result of my mother or stepfather's cultural influence. During my childhood I recall music wasn't played at home by my mother on the radio when I was living there. She also told me

'Terry doesn't like it'. I'm told he mellowed in later years and my mother said he did like music, contrasting with what he told me.

Like all young kids of my age, I had the smallest of transistor radios and soaked up the music on Radio Luxembourg late into the night underneath the bed blankets.

My mother drove all kinds of vehicles during the war, including lorries when in the army but afterwards while she was married to Terry she only drove in an emergency. Strange again.

About the music, it may have been that my stepdad Terry, especially when I was a teenager going out and performing music, disliked it because he knew where my gift had come from. My mother must surely have told him about Syd's abilities, though Syd I'm certain was a taboo topic of conversation between them during their marriage unless of course the pair were arguing.

My musical gift had come courtesy of the unspoken one, the ghost who haunted Terry and Judy's relationship from time to time and sometimes turning it rocky. Syd's ghost always around. Of course, music was one reason my mum got together with my dad. To Terry I was a permanent reminder that Syd had existed though he had tried to shut him out.

My mother told me that Terry was jealous of her previous relationship with Syd and insisted she put the past behind her by burning all photographs of Syd.

But Terry started the marriage between himself and Judy with a poor hand because when they married, she didn't love him.

My mother even told me in a letter when we were corresponding with her in her 90's that I had chosen Terry for her. I had been a babe in arms but nevertheless had reached out to him in making a choice between two men vying for her attention. My outstretched arms to Terry were enough for her to make her decision.

CHAPTER SEVEN

MUM AND DAD IN DIFFERENT HOSPITALS AT THE SAME TIME...

My late father Syd was with my mum to be at home in the West Midlands when her waters broke, and she realised she had to be taken quickly to the hospital in readiness for my birth. A taxi was needed and fast.

Syd left the house to go to a telephone box to call for one and Judy waited and waited, but Syd didn't return.

She had no idea why the delay or what was happening and my time of arrival in this world was imminent.

In the end, it was Syd's dad who took Judy to hospital. Now both she and my grandad-to-be were concerned about Syd's absence. Where was he? He seemed to have vanished.

Syd had been weak and poorly for some time as the cancer ate away at his insides and on his way to the telephone box he had collapsed in the street.

He had then been taken by ambulance to hospital.

Both my mum and dad were now in different hospitals in Birmingham as my mother gave birth to me.

No, you couldn't make it up!

This tragic outcome was related to me by my mother in one of her later, in fact very late letters to me.

My mother's life at that stage was never straight forward and now having been born I was incorporated into this chaotic situation caused by that atomic bomb!

Syd came out of hospital. He had expressed a wish to die at home and he did, aged just 26.

With Syd gone I was still a babe in arms.

After my mother and I were reunited on Facebook and in one of the letter's my mother wrote me to broaden my knowledge of what went on in my past she took me back to a time not that long after my father's death.

Mother had taken in two lodgers at her house in Wednesbury, Staffordshire – the house she and Syd were going to live in – and one of these men was Terry.

And my mother's memory or the indication in the letter I received was that both of those lodgers were attracted to her and that perhaps she had a choice which she should 'take on'.

In my mother's apologetic letter following one of our Facebook disagreements, she explained that I was a baby held in her arms when she faced two men standing in front of her.

And I was to outstretch my arms towards Terry, this she then interpreted as a sign that I was choosing Terry for her.

This suggestion has a hint of Walt Disney romance about it. As a journalist I'd have written the headline: 'BABY CHOOSES NEXT DAD'.

My interpretation of what she did on this historic occasion was to cannily play the avoidance card. She hadn't chosen Terry

I had. She was a mere onlooker as she watched Terry and I bond leaving the other lodger to ride off into the sunset.

Her apparent version was that she had only complied with my wish by accepting Terry. It was therefore pure and simple sacrifice on her part. She selected him after my intervention on her behalf. In her eyes I had clearly made my recommendation.

Ever after, it surely can't have been the case, can it, that I took the blame for every ensuing argument she and Terry had, and they had many – for me having made the wrong choice of suitor for her? Did she at times wish I had chosen the other lodger? I am only joking, I think!

During my childhood I always felt mum sounded and played the martyr to great effect, but I never understood why or knew the circumstances behind it.

If ever she felt that I had done something wrong, then the prelude too whatever else she was going to accuse me of was always: "After all that I've done for you in my life…" She weighed me down with guilt. It certainly taught me to keep quiet and not to upset or offend someone who had made so much sacrifice for me, even though I was unaware of the sacrifices that she had made because she hadn't told me what they were.

Mine was a life lived scrambling in the dark! No clues.

Following the Facebook interchange and the death of my mother my sister asked me if I remembered the time when we were children when my dad and mum were arguing and a butter knife was thrown. Liz told me mum was packing her suitcase and: "She was going to leave us, but take you with her?"

That would have left Terry behind to look after my stepbrother and sister, the children of their coupling. My mother having compartmentalised her life, would have walked away from the marriage to Terry with me, Syd's child.

Make of that what you will, a division, a deep schism in the ranks perhaps. At times of crisis my mother I think went back to the time when she faced her worst crisis, when she was going to kill us. A time when it was only, she and I against the world, as it had been when Syd tragically died. If she had coped with what had happened then, she could cope with anything, she must have believed.

I always considered my story was too complex to write about. I was certainly wrestling throughout my life with unexpressed feelings, and I was lost for words that matched to tell how I felt. I just couldn't explain all the things that happened until later in life when it all finally started falling into place.

I'd been trying all my life to complete my jigsaw puzzle with too many missing pieces.

On the positive side, thank God, like Syd, I had been gifted with a songwriter's ability to enable me to practice what I never realised was a kind of self-therapy.

From an early age I wanted to write the saddest of all songs. I wanted to touch other people with the hurt and loneliness that I felt inside and could only get out myself through music.

I considered a song was only any good if it made people cry and made them feel empathetic with how I was feeling. If it put people in touch with their emotions, then it would be a job well done.

I wanted to reach out to those who felt as I did, trapped inside without words to say how they felt or thought. I guessed there were millions of us at that time suffering quietly in misery especially as politics in this country never seemed to offer much to take us out of the mire. Most the time politicians led us from one crisis to another, making decisions we the ordinary folk had no say or control over. Nothing changes.

Paradoxically, I did enjoy the misery I was feeling because it released in me repressed emotions. The finished songs, words and music were an escape to elation as well as giving me a sense of accomplishment.

It was my best and only way for my emotions to be heard. When the music business started showing an interest in my music, I was only half interested though many companies expressed great interest and they saw a great deal of money to be made from them.

I was only half interested because these songs were part of me, they were personal. Too personal to give to anyone or sell. I was extremely reluctant to let them go to market least they be altered or spoiled. My songs had the significance to me of babies. I took great care of them. Not only that but I was aware the music business would lead me away from my greatest joy the writing of music. I would have less time to do it. Every musician who signs a deal eventually realises the business side of music is a poison chalice.

CHAPTER EIGHT

HATE MAIL

It was after I left home as a young man of 19, that I received the destructive hate mail from my mother.

She and I had never spoken heart to heart. Feelings were buried. She was full of secrets. As I said, it led to our 50-year estrangement.

Only now have I made sense of my past by making sense of hers as she finally laid out her truths aged 91.

My mother before meeting Syd had escaped a difficult childhood upbringing during which both her parents died. Let her tell you as the 91-year-old who wrote these messages sent to me on Facebook. She was enlightening me about the past she had kept hidden.

'I didn't have a good childhood my mum had eleven babies in thirteen years only eight lived then one died. When I was five my dad had TB (tuberculosis). Mum died at 39, dad at 40. There were five kids and me all boys me being the only girl I had most of the housework to do! I was kept off school to look after my dad and the boys. I didn't go.

'I didn't go to school until I was nearly twelve. Then they put us all with foster parents. I was abused by my foster father then couldn't take it anymore and at sixteen and a half I ran off to join the RNG. For the first time I had new clothes and I paid for them. My foster mother tried to get me returned but my commanding officer told her I belonged to the army.'

Note – know the numbers don't add up but these are my mother's words.

There you have it, in just a couple of paragraphs, an insight into what a dire childhood my mother experienced. What with assuming the responsibilities of an adult when she was a child herself, the alleged abuse from her foster father and later losing Syd to cancer, is it any wonder that without counselling she had toughed it out to become at times the strong but contrary woman she could be. She must have built a defence system inside of her as secure as Fort Knox to avoid further hurt.

What person given her circumstances would not have wanted to leave the past behind? She had experienced a catalogue of misery.

After the loss of Syd, she was a young woman with a baby making a fresh start for herself from Ground Zero. My question is this, was it possible for someone to leave behind such a traumatic past, as was her intention, and the past not affect her future behaviour? How on earth did she contain and manage that hurt especially with repeating sad or awful haunting memories – and at the expense of what did she manage it?

Not many secrets go through life untold.

It would be naïve to think that those memories, those feelings she locked away did not shape her decisions or effect those around her. I believe the rawness of her past was always with her having never properly dealt with how she felt and why. I think that state existed even up to her death and of course it did have a drastic and negative outcome on our relationship.

Those repressed, secret memories of my mother's, were why while I was growing up, my mother was incapable of talking to me, or anyone else in the family at that time, intimately about her feelings. She may well have been wanting to spare me the gory details of her own past, but equally as harmful as it turned out for me was her hiding of the truth and the shutting down of her true feelings and emotions.

When she committed herself to her second marriage to Terry, she hadn't loved him and Syd was the ghost she still loved, and this she had told to my siblings later in life too.

Already she had battened down the hatches emotionally. That emptiness inside that she must have felt at times, I experienced too. I learned from her how to block off feelings and not to speak of my own emotions.

Parents can never truly understand how much or how little their children's behaviour is shaped by them. These days there is a name for it when parents get it wrong. Childhood Emotional Neglect or CEN. Some parenting damages children and parents don't even realise what it is they are doing or have done wrong. Some parents imagine they are doing everything right in their child's upbringing but instead a child or children are rendered detached from love and support, emotionally bereft, disturbed or left with unanswered questions that still rear their head in adulthood.

I was approaching 20 when I cheerfully and with no regret left home immediately to get married. After I had left home, whenever my mother had a gripe about me, she would never pick up a phone or meet up to talk it out instead, and especially after I left my marriage, she wrote me what I considered the poisonous letters.

She wrote with razor attacking sharpness and told me I was 'no son of hers' and 'You will die in the gutter'.

The anger she felt while writing was illustrated by her underlining of key words usually twice in bold biro. using such force that it was a good job she used quality Basildon Bond paper otherwise the pen would have ripped through the paper!

I came to dread and hate those letters, which I understand she kept on writing to others long after I had made myself scarce. The cruelty of her words made up my mind for me. With no knowledge of her upbringing or young adulthood I had no reason to think that perhaps these were the actions of a damaged woman.

At the time I viewed her vindictiveness as a form of abuse. Maybe then, like Terry, I too was competing with the ghost of Syd. Her Syd would never behave as I did. I had not only let her down but Syd too? Mum also liked to control things.

I decided that my mother was no good for me and I was better off without her. I cut her off as deliberately as she had decided to have nothing to do with me.

74

This was the stand-off that lasted more than 50 years.

Long, long ago she had cut Syd out of her life, but had salvaged for herself memories, sweet memories of love and dark memories of loss running deep, but these were for her own private consumption, no-one else's. She had cut Syd's side of the family out of her life when she decided to move on and neither would she until really late in life have any further contact with her own large family in Bolton. She may have been incapable emotionally of building bridges with others and that would not have surprised me. Maybe she didn't have the words to describe the repressed emotions she felt swirling inside of her. I know that feeling myself.

I had no idea why she did abandon relationships, why she left never to look back. She most likely wouldn't have known how to repair them. For a long time, I didn't know how to do that either. I had never learned. I understand now why she was the way she was.

I was informed by her when I was 10 years old that the man who I thought was my father Terry was in fact was not my father.

She told me in a sentence in what can best be described as an ambush.

"Terry is not your dad," she said after she came up to my bedroom and we were alone.

I remember to this day uttering my child's reply, perhaps by saying the only thing that could be said in those circumstances. I expressed denial saying: "But he is my dad."

Hearing this family revelation was a bolt out of the blue. I wasn't even sat down. I was stood up. These days you'd have a therapist on hand – or maybe two or three on stand-by for something quite as traumatic.

Having heard my response with my own five words uttered in shocked reply, my mother spun on her heels and left my bedroom at speed. I heard her bolting fast down the stairs. It was if she was running away. She was. She was running away from telling me anymore. It was job done she must have thought.

It had been necessary for the child to know that the man he thought was his father wasn't really and was in fact only his stepdad. She had done her duty telling me this. But that was it. That wasn't the start point, it was the finish. She never elaborated. Never opened further discussion. Were there any questions that I wanted to ask she might have asked me? It might have been a good start point from which to learn more. But that wasn't to be a start point to learn more. The door was locked tight on the subject and never while I was at home was the subject raised again. That was my introduction to my father's ghost.

Terry in all our time together never spoke about meeting my mother, or about my father or even my adoption. He never spoke of why he had adopted me or of the adoption itself. He never told me how he felt about me. He never expressed his love for me, though he might have felt it, but who knows? My mother insisted that he did love me. Should it be necessary to guess if you are loved when you are a child? Doesn't when a parent says they love you it makes you feel just a little bit special? Doesn't it make you feel emotionally secure and supported? But he was another, not capable of speaking of his own emotions. His were probably bottled too. Men of his era it is said, didn't express emotion they were regarded as the tougher gender as a result, but even as a child I thought it strange and lacking that people had to feel so strongly about stuff but had no means to tell anyone about it. To me it still is extraordinary that things that needed saying in the various houses where we lived never were.

My brother and sister Liz and Chris, Terry's children by Judy, were told of my background much later, after I'd left home, that I had been adopted. They were taken aside to be enlightened, maintaining that secrecy again. I don't know if Terry and Judy both did the telling and they were telling the same story or whether it was just my mother controlling the agenda.

I wonder with hindsight why they could not have held a family gathering so that we could all share the truth together and talk about it, with me included so that I was able to know everyone's reaction? These were the days before inclusivity. Was this my mother's continued way of controlling the truth, telling it to one, one way and to another in another way, keeping control of it. It worked that way for her.

My mother anyway preferred her own version of the truth or her own outlook on things, to anyone else's.

Giving her the benefit of the doubt, she was creative with the truth. Some of the things she told me in my early years which I later raised with her she denied ever saying. Secrecy had cloaked everything. Syd was whispered about, and my brother and sister were probably told I knew all about Syd and his background already. But I didn't. I much, much, later discovered they knew more than me or had conflicting stories to my own. What did they ask and what replies did they get from my mother? My mother would have chosen in my absence to represent my views, interpret my reaction etc. I never spoke for myself.

I knew I was viewed by her in a bad light, but I didn't care. That umbilical cord was cut. To this day with my mother now having passed our family might still not be singing from the same hymn sheet, not knowing the same things. It is not paranoid to think that we might know secrets about one another that are untrue because my mum led the whispering propaganda operation.

To learn the history or truth of what has happened in a family it takes a tremendous amount of courage and stamina, it involves sifting through clues, knocking down of walls, co-operation with others, examination or interpretation of behavioural patterns of family members, unravelling of long held beliefs and the unravelling too even of what we held once as precious truths.

The levee can only take so much before it bursts. Truth will out, hopefully!

After breaking the news that my father was not my father in my bedroom, my mother didn't brooch the subject again. I might have imagined it hadn't happened. It seemed unreal. Hadn't there been more she wanted or needed to say in that moment too free herself further? I wasn't sure who my real father was or even where he was, if he was alive or not because he hadn't been around to visit me, and I was now ten. I hadn't been introduced to him. Was he dead or alive? He was unspoken of. Was he a serial killer? Did we not speak his name out of shame?

A child doesn't easily ask difficult or awkward questions of a parent especially when they sense or know that no-one really wants to sit down and elaborate. Neither Terry or Judy did. I only began to discover more about my early background and my real father in later life. Everything comes to those who wait.

CHAPTER NINE

SCAREDY CAT USES SCHOOL PRESS TO BEAT TEACHER BULLY

Who can blame a boy for being a Scaredy Cat when he is being bullied at school by a teacher. That happened to me. I thought I'd have to take this bloke's dislike and insults for at least another two years of my school life, until remarkably that teacher opened his mouth to make the biggest tongue slip of his life. When he did, I was then able as a 14-year-old to practise for the first time the journalism that demonstrates the power of the press.

My woodwork teacher was my persecutor at school. He made my life a misery. I was afraid of him. He had groomed me that way with his constant picking on me. Woodwork teachers in my era could be a little over the top as masculine specimens if not downright sadistic. This one was hairy armed though as small as Hitler or Mussolini and always had his sleeves rolled up to show off those symbolic arms while attired in his working kit of brown overalls.

Those muscles of his had been honed by knocking nails into or sawing wood, not pursuits I was the slightest bit interested in. At my previous school where every teacher used canes on pupils, he would have been in his element. At this school only the headmaster now had permission to brandish that instrument of torture and was entitled to do so putting a pupil whose behaviour was off the scale straight with a good whacking usually with boys it was on the seat of the pants.

I was a slim, weedy boy. Nothing you can do about that. I looked a perfect foil for a bully. However, I was not without spunk. I was built perfectly for running and had the guts to match. I was running longer and longer distances, but Mr Woodwork didn't regard me as a tough guy but someone to exploit to show off his own manliness. God, he was pathetic. I got bullied by this nerd of a teacher during times when there was no protection against his like. Abuse of power. He gave me a dread of attending woodwork lessons.

A few times unbeknown to my parents, who I didn't dare tell of my predicament because of dire communication problems at home, I did skive off school and rode around the countryside on my bicycle instead.

Mr Woodwork always strode manfully into the classroom. He owned the space around him, but the greedy sod wanted my space too. He walked chest puffed out proudly and his hair heavily plastered down with hair cream. An aggressive snarl was never far from his face when talking down certain boys. He laughed at his own jokes, these sarcastic, considered the lowest form of wit. He surrounded himself with young boy sycophants. These were my classmates who most of them he had convinced that their ambitions should be to become woodwork teachers. Most went on to fail 'A' level woodwork. Anyway, in class they laughed along with him and formed themselves quickly into circles around him when he demanded it. "Form a circle, boys," he would command. He loved to be the centre of attention and he'd stand in the middle. Typically, one day he stood me up in front of the class during a technical drawing lesson and yelled: "Boy. What do you intend doing when you leave this school?"

It came out the blue. He was intent on having another pop at me. I had been sat there minding my own business but probably doodling.

He was out to intimidate and very loudly and sarcastically. He was about to point out to everyone in my class that I was the kind of boy he not only did not like, as I was relatively quiet, skinny and not at all hairy armed, but that I was destined too for life's scrapheap without his woodwork and technical drawing skills.

"Stand up, boy," he ordered me. I did. My throat went dry.

"Well, boy what will you do when you leave this school…"

I replied: "I want to work on a newspaper, Sir."

"Delivering them no doubt," he replied with his hands on his hips and throwing back his head, his 'joke' causing gales of laughter at my expense from all the boys – the girls were occupied doing domestic science in another classroom while we learned the boys' skills to equip us for life.

It was no funny joke that the woodwork teacher had cracked but the traitorous snides' around me laughed betraying any friendship or loyalty they might have thought they owed me.

They did it so Mr Woodwork would continue picking on me because that meant he would not start torturing one of them instead.

However, I should be grateful to that low life of a teacher, that disgrace to his profession from the bottom of my heart for educating me just how powerful the press was as a tool to rescue the underdog.

One day in the lunchtime school canteen Mr Woodwork was prowling and cracking his whip on staff dinner duty and he brazenly told more than 150 pupils in the dining hall. "My dog has better table manners than you lot."

Oh yes?

Now the school at the time was blessed with a newspaper called *Rendezvous* and I contributed.

I did a fortnightly fictional story called '*The Kids of County Blinkshire*' which was about the anarchic pupils who ran roughshod over the teachers. I was the JK Rowling of my school and of my time. Now I was about to ditch my reputation as Clark Kent and become instead… superman.

I did not feel offended by what Mr Woodwork had claimed – that his dog had better table manners than me and the rest of the young people eating in the school canteen, but I thought he should be made to stand by his statement and prove to us that his dog was that special and could teach us how to eat properly. I wanted to see if his dog – which we had seen sight of and of course it was a dangerous looking Alsatian – could handle cutlery using its paws better than those amongst us who were the worst at handling utensils utilising fingers in the school canteen.

I submitted a story to *Rendezvous* challenging Mr Woodwork to produce his dog in the canteen so we could all see if it lived up to up his billing as the dog with the best table manners of any dog, possibly in the world.

If it could live up to its billing it belonged not as Mr Woodwork's pet but in a big top at a circus.

That dog had lost its way stuck in Mr Woodwork's kitchen eating bones with its knife and fork when it could be on TV giving demonstrations. After this story made headlines, there would be a case for all dogs to be educated in table manners and to start using knives forks and spoons. All dogs would follow where this highly civilised Alsatian was leading.

I submitted this piece of constructive reporting to our school newspaper, and it led to merry hell breaking out.

It became clear that Mr Woodwork wasn't as popular as he thought he was, especially with fellow teachers who probably saw through his masculine pomposity and silly posing.

Some teachers were delighted that the alpha male Mr Woodwork was being challenged to show us his performing Alsatian, the one with the perfect table manners.

One teacher especially, the bearded editor of Rendezvous, congratulated me on having a pop at Mr Woodwork's assertion and said it was my right to have my story published though Mr Woodwork he said, had been told and had gone green around the gills. He didn't want my article published in Rendezvous. But freedom of the press was what mattered most not the reputation of the woodwork teacher the editor told me. Good man.

My English teacher Mr Peter Price who was my great inspiration at school and who encouraged me to write, became my intermediator and told me Mr Woodwork now wanted a pow wow with me.

What followed was a scene I had only once seen replicated on the western film High Noon. I met Mr Woodwork in an empty tech drawing room one lunchtime, and he was, err very different towards me. He even had his sleeves drawn down over his hairy arms. That was almost like seeing a flagpole with the flag at half-mast.

He asked very politely, as if suddenly I had become his best mate, if I would withdraw my story. He was no longer alpha or being bombastic with me. He wasn't insulting. He was worried that the national newspapers would get hold of the story if Rendezvous published it and it would make him look an idiot.

I noticed his consideration was only for himself. He had no thoughts for the new career his dog might miss if my story was withdrawn. Fame in a new town beckoned for that clever dog. Performances in a circus big top but more importantly I thought that even the dog would be grateful to me for freeing him from the clutches of Mr Woodwork. Imagine living with a bombastic sourpuss like him?

My adversary was placatory. As my tech drawing was so poor, he said he would give me private lessons and bring me up to speed. What? I almost convulsed. I hated technical drawing. He thought everybody should love technical drawing because he taught it. I didn't want to do more of it I wanted less or even better none of it. Now he was on the ropes and trying to negotiate a deal. He was desperate. He hated me before, but now he was reduced to begging.

I realised I could make a deal that would suit my purposes. I could get him off my back with some smart thinking, clever negotiating. Brain could beat brawn. The pen was mightier than the sword.

I told him I wanted nothing more to do with his woodwork or technical drawing classes. I wasn't cut out for the subjects, I told him. I just wasn't interested but I wanted him off my back. He agreed and he never did trouble me again. I had gone back to the editor after my pow wow and told him I was letting Mr Woodwork off the hook. The editor smiled. It was still the power of the press that had done it! He knew it and so did I.

The woodwork teacher must have then continued to hate my guts though because this scrawny kid had not only got one over on him but always defeated his house runners in the school cross country championship.

That was my first experience of using the power of the press. It felt good. Very good. I was to use it to great effect during my long career in journalism much of the time fighting the causes of underdogs.

I suppose Mr Woodwork might have been said to have got his revenge in another sense because I scored the lowest possible grade in woodwork in my GCE exam. I was proud of it.

The headmaster going through my results with me said: "A grade 9 for woodwork. I've never known anyone score as low as that before."

I thanked Mr Woodwork's Alsatian for my low mark. That Grade 9 was my badge of honour.

Incidentally, my headmaster had always shown himself concerned for my educational welfare. His overall comment on my performance in the year before my GCE exams was: "Alan should pay more attention to things like getting his hair cut."

I think I rankled the headmaster.

He was a firm believer in democracy and introduced voting amongst the boys and girls to select Head Boy and Head Girl.

I was elected head boy. Then I also won elections for school sports captain, house captain and house sport captain.

With my long hair and my refusal to wear a necktie and to always wear trainers and not shoes (everybody wore shoes at the time), I wasn't the headmaster's choice of an example for other pupils to follow.

But he did come into class once though and conceded to my fellow classmates: "Charnley will one day be elected Mayor of Rotherham with his track record of election victories."

He got that wrong.

CHAPTER TEN

GROWING UP IN THE DARK

There was nobody of any consequence or maturity to keep a check on my mother or her actions as I was growing up as a lad. Anyone trying would have got short thrift from her had they tried. It was a matriarchal home and run like clockwork. She was blinkered and high energised. You might have described her as a force of nature, but even nature is not on its best behaviour all the time.

As a child, I was short of relatives, other adult role models. I accepted it as normal that we had no extended family with whom there could be a closeness or affinity. I didn't know what nephews and nieces were until I was well into my late 20's not having met or mixed with any.

At school when I was required through religion to select a godfather for confirmation into the Catholic Church, other children in my class had ready-made family or friends to select from. My parents had no-one to call upon, so it was my schoolteacher who was a nice, tall bloke with glasses, but a stranger to me and of whom I knew nothing, who was handed the job.

He could have been a devil worshipper, but he became my godfather in a church ceremony. That role for him, where he made a pledge to keep a sharp eye on my spiritual welfare for a lifetime, lasted as long as the ceremony itself did. Where he went after the 'ceremony' I have no idea! All I know is that he was a fleeting link with myself and God. Mr Sanderson was his name. He'll be in heaven himself by now and will have been ticked off by God for leaving me in his absence more susceptible to Satan's overtures.

With hindsight, judging from the later Basildon Bond Exocet letters my mother sent me, she might have been repeating on me the type of ticking offs she herself had received during her earlier life, maybe from her foster parents. Maybe they wrote to her ordering her to come home after she had run off to the army with a warning she would die in the gutter if she didn't.

That threat didn't work with her. It didn't work either on me.

Lesson. We all learn our behaviours good or bad from someone.

She was perhaps insecure and felt aloneness in what at first anyway had been on her part a loveless marriage. She had made a sacrifice and had that sacrifice been made just for me so that I could grow up in a traditional family? How did she feel as I was growing up and when I felt the need to express my independence and leave home, somewhat abruptly? Did she feel it was a betrayal for me to leave after all she had done for me? Could I ever do enough of what she might have expected of me?

Sooner rather than later I felt the need for independence and to lose the feeling of claustrophobia I felt living at home.

By the time I was a young man I just felt I had to make some sense of myself, and she was no help. I needed to put distance between us. At home I had likened my position anyway to that of a cuckoo in the nest.

I didn't miss my mother when I left home because there was nothing to miss. There had been a rigorous discipline imposed at home during my childhood that was of it time and was supposed to do us children good, and in some respects it did, but to my way of thinking it was never complemented by outward signs of love or reason or explanation. It shaped up at times more like a military camp. Maybe the pair of them ran the house as they did the shoe shop? I worked at that shoe shop for a time as a schoolboy on Saturdays and holidays and that too was very regimented with Terry barking at his female staff impatiently most of the time addressing them as 'Miss' with a snarl. My mother ran around like a blue-arsed fly upstairs instructing her team of women. Give them credit though for hard work and discipline.

After I had left home my mum was left with the family of four – she and Terry's children but when she visited me alone once, at my house, the one with the old Methodist church piano, and for the only time when she did so alone with the intention of speaking to me, she uncharacteristically spilled out her unhappiness.

She wanted to be free again, she told me, as free as she had been in the army. She wished to be, she said, like a gypsy, able to go and live anywhere, at any time she chose. Her relationship with Terry was not all it could be for her, she said. She spoke of her love for children and how her ideal would be working in a children's home.

FACING SURGERY? DON'T BE A SCAREDY CAT

Of course, when my children came along, her grandchildren, that fulfilled her craving. On that day she spoke to me, with hindsight she'd have been better off speaking to a therapist. I admit I was resentful of her on this occasion as we hadn't communicated all through our lives, now she was spilling this personal information about herself. I was pent up with frustration unable to know where to start addressing my own issues with her myself. She never had asked me how I was feeling. I was as helpful though as I could have been that day. She wanted to know how to deal with how she felt. I suggested she wrote about it to make sense of it. She did start a book which my brother now tells me he has. He is being kind he says by not showing it to me because of the unkind, but possibly worse things my mother wrote about me in the back pages of it. Her poison words back to haunt me even after her death.

I figured or feared she would always write me a last letter of hate before her death. I had vowed never to open it. I'd know if it was from her and not to open it. It would be written on Basildon Bond product. Fortunately, she and I resolved our differences, but the unread horrid last thoughts of Judy linger there for me to read one day. I'm not going to bother.

When I left my marriage, my wife and kids, after 11 years after marrying as a 19-years-old, her letters to me were vile, but she never asked why I had split from my wife, or how I felt. We never met to discuss it. I was alone with my feelings and with no-one to discuss my break-up. I didn't make sense of it. I did what she did. I buried it and decided to get on with life. I drank a lot too. Society then preached what was best for the children if a couple broke up was what they called a 'clean break' by the couple. That's what I did. Marriage hadn't solved any of the internal problems I wrestled with. I had worked hard and been responsible, but I still felt empty inside. Help and advice wasn't around in those days as much as it is today to untangle the mess that sometimes accumulates in our heads. These days there must be a ratio of one psychotherapist available for every person in the UK.

Everybody seem to be a psychotherapist in the town where I now live and prior to that most I have come across were patients themselves.

What I did in my era was to do what my mother did in hers. You sorted yourself out alone.

I hadn't realised it at the time, but now I had done exactly what she had done in all her early life's situations. I walked away without explanation. I did that because I didn't have the words to say how I was feeling. I did what most people were advised to do then – but I'd also inherited her modus operandum.

During my marriage, I had been writing miserable songs on my piano about how I was feeling for not months but years. I felt I was down a cul-de-sac and going nowhere. I'd taken a wrong turning. I hoped my wife would pick up my vibe. She probably just liked the sad songs. She didn't ask why the songs were miserable and we never had the conversation about them or about us, if of course it had been possible to have a conversation with me at that time. It hadn't been possible for me at any stage to talk about my emotions with my mother, so I lacked practise. I was a clam. It wasn't a bad marriage but despite all the emotional content I put into songs about breaking up and making up etc. in reality I was rather an emotional cripple in practical terms.

I was painted as a villain in the letters my mother sent after I left home, but I was a lost soul. With the coast clear and me having left my home, she then in one of her Facebook messages towards the end of her days told me – and I knew that she viewed it this way before informing me – "When you left, I got the kids."

She hadn't after all needed to go and work in that children's home.

If I had returned to my marital home, repaired things with my wife, my mother wouldn't have had the access to the kids she had. You see I wanted to tell her not to come to the house as often as she did uninvited and to be respectful and call first to see if it was convenient. It was not only the polite thing to do but then I would not have seen her as so pushy. I didn't want her bringing along with her either the multiple provisions that might have fed an African nation.

I didn't want to be bought. I wanted my independence from her. We didn't need food buying or fetching. I was doing alright. Better than alright, but she was still a running sore. I didn't want her suffocating parenting of me to rub off on my kids. It still was rubbing off on me.

I was very close to telling her but who was going to see it my way, my wife? Understandably she thought my mum wonderful and welcomed the provisions. Mind you, my wife didn't know how much my past had affected me and then again neither did I know as much about it as I know now so I couldn't have explained to her how I felt.

Not many people could have had the same mother and son relationship in my early years as we did, given our dreadful circumstances.

I didn't have the words to explain how I was feeling at the time of my marriage split. There was too much going on in my head that I couldn't make sense of. I did what my mother had taught me. I just blocked off my feelings. I went and got on with life.

But back to my childhood aged 12 or more, and every Thursday I used to arrive home late afternoon when my mother who worked in a shoe shop five days a week took her day off. It was we knew her bungalow cleaning day. My stepfather was the manager of the shoe shop. In truth, she was the boss, he was the manager, perhaps in name only at least that was the way she once told it to me.

On Thursdays, mother used to spend the whole day cleaning our bungalow home from top to bottom, every nook and cranny. When I arrived home late afternoon from school, she would be in a rage and complain loudly about all the work it had been necessary to do. Then she'd lose her temper completely and take exception to the state of my room. She'd then set about me with her bony fists on the pretext that my room was the messiest and most untidy. It was hardly that; she would never have allowed it to decay to the extent that she made out. Thursday to Thursday didn't leave me much time anyway to turn my bedroom into an infested, grubby disaster zone. She was brim full of frustration and hate. She squeaked and squealed taking out whatever frustrations these were of hers out upon me.

Mother's control extended to forbidding us children from pinning up football posters on the bedroom wall. Other children in families could do it and have posters of pop stars or footballers but she tore mine down. The bedroom had to be kept pristine, maybe she was echoing a drill sergeant who had given her grief while she was in the army. Had she been hauled over the coals, criticised for her standard of cleanliness while she'd been in the ranks? Who knows where this deep-seated angst came from?

While she rained blows on me for my alleged untidiness, I used to be on the bed with my hands protectively covering my head. She would scream and whimper in anger. I remember clearly those sounds she made. Animalistic. She went berserk. I had a similar woman schoolteacher, a bony thin bespectacled fervent Catholic at my primary school, a spinster old before her time who used to jab me on the head with a biro. Madness prevailed, in those days.

My stepfather Terry would arrive home at the bungalow on Thursdays a few hours later having taxied my brother and sister home from their schools in the city and they'd all be no wiser about what had happened to me. There was no-one for me to tell even if I had desired to do so. The thing was in those days you had to nobly accept punishment for your 'sins' and not complain. It was character building. A bashing was a common punishment for the wayward child. It was important a child was disciplined to learn the errors of their ways.

Although the Second World War had finished many of the army disciplines of that time seemed to have slipped into civilian life! It was considered less male, a weakness and feeble to complain. Punishment was always deserved and justified.

I got struck at school by teachers at various schools who used rulers, canes or straps and I never reported that treatment back home because teachers in those days, some clearly identifiable as sadists, had an entitlement or a legal 'cover', to practice their dark arts. Schools in my day were run by the strict laws of the jungle. The boys at my first secondary school – a 'sink' school with that terminology going nowhere near to summing up its bleak awfulness and poor standard of education – took it in turns to own up to misbehaviours so that innocent lads shared the cane with the guilty. Crazy! That school was so bad it was closed for good a year after I had arrived, and I transferred to a new school.

My mother always used to be warning my stepfather: "Keep your hands off him." She was referring to me.

I think if Terry took exception to my behaviour he had to go through the correct channel. If he wanted to censure me then mother was that channel. I reckon early in the relationship that mother had made this agreement that as I was Syd's kid and not his, therefore she would administer any punishment that they as a couple felt I was deserving of.

As usual I was blithely unaware of the reasons for my mother's switchblade moods. There were times when she'd burst into my room while I was playing innocently and shout at me that I was 'coming between' her and Terry.

What?

Other times, she would hurry into my room, once again for no apparent reason and would grab hold of me and hug me tightly professing how much she loved me and how I was her favourite child out of three of us because I was 'special'. That I later termed as 'smother love'. I didn't understand what was going on at the time, and because you are confused and don't, you don't forget either. It was like being loved or not at the flick of some switch inside her head. I never knew what was coming next.

Life went on with Terry spending most of his time in the garages of any new properties we moved to live in. He'd don his dark blue overalls and into the garage he would vanish for hours upon end. He might have lived in his garages. His head was always in a car bonnet. As a child I could never figure how he could have kept himself so occupied doing what he did. I was told he took engines apart and then put them back together.

He did invite me into his garage once and started telling me how the combustion engine worked, but he could see there was no enthusiasm on my part. I just wasn't practical in that way.

But it's funny what you remember as a child. That day that was supposed to be my garage initiation he told me that my mum had told him that they were destined to meet, but that he didn't believe in that sort of thing. Mum maybe did believe it was destiny and he was the rescue ship that came along when she and I were drowning.

If Terry left the garage, it was to decorate or revamp the houses or bungalows where we lived. He would complete an in-house project until everything looked brand spanking new, and then sometimes very soon after he would replace it or redo it.

Our house maintenance was conducted like the painting of the Forth Bridge. It was well known that workmen who finished painting the Firth Bridge, because the bridge was so long immediately had to start repainting from the beginning again and straight away. Once Terry had painted or decorated to the end of a house he would begin again, maybe at the request of my mother. This was a carbon copy of my mother's housework behaviour. She was tied, as I said, to housework, continuous motion like a hamster is to a wheel in a cage. She rushed at it, always rushing and as a song of that period pointed out, played on radio most of the time: 'a girl's work is never done...'.

My mum and dad never socialised with friends while I was at living home. I'm not sure they ever had friends. I don't ever recall friends visiting. I do remember however them interviewing a string of babysitters for us, but they were all so bad that as the oldest child I ended up babysitting illegally for my younger sister and brother from the age of around 11 years old, every Saturday and on school holidays when both parents were at work. I didn't get paid and anyway would not have been so brash as to ask.

One of our babysitters, an old woman, having sailed through her interview with my parents, on taking up her post had then lectured us about the evils of Christmas, and another was a Jehovah's witness who my parents found out was indoctrinating us. They had both been employed at first, and separately of course as 'nice people' but sacked when their respective proclivities and inner motives were revealed. They were then considered as the next worst thing to child snatchers.

Meanwhile Terry always built his high fences outside and around the properties wherever we lived. No-one could see in, and we couldn't see out. He loved his cowboy films did Terry,

John Wayne and western library books and our house always resembled the outside of Fort Apache. Terry and Judy lived in one another's pockets living and working together, well almost! Terry's bolthole of course was his garage, and he was the boss on the downstairs floor of the shoe shop while my mother policed the upstairs. They kept to their lines of demarcation just as we three children did when we had to make a civilised line to have our daily dose of cod and liver oil.

I don't attach blame to my mother for what she did or who she had become after learning about her own hard times. The purpose of my putting words to paper was to understand my fractured past life more fully. It is like putting together a jigsaw puzzle for which I now have more pieces. I'll never have them all. This is the best I can do. I want to put the past in its place, behind me. It lingered too long in a messy jumble at the forefront of my mind. There must be countless others out there with unknown mothers or fathers who wish they knew more about family than they have ever been told. It impacts greatly not to know.

Mother was forged in her own time by some horrendous circumstances that prevailed in her early life including poverty. While messaging on Facebook she told me of the times when as a girl she went scavenging on the street after the market had left for the day for any discarded fruit or vegetables so her family could eat.

We are all forged by how we deal with our own very differing circumstances. Having spent time re-uniting with her on Facebook I wished her no ill will. I just wished we could have talked more about what really mattered when I was a kid, a teenager or as a young adult, when she was the adult parent.

The truth is that it is probably rare to find any adult is ever properly prepared or equipped for parenthood. We make it up as we go along. Parenthood sneaks up upon us young adults and in my case, it was sooner rather than later because I hadn't worn a condom because my adopted religion told me it was sinful to prevent procreation. The more the merrier, my faith Roman Catholicism decreed.

Parenthood in my day happened and the expectation was that you tied the knot with someone to do the decent thing and to give a baby a surname, which in my case wasn't really my surname anyway, not that I knew that back then!

I married because I was looking for love, but I may not have been very good at recognising it when it came along.

Some adults stubbornly remain kids even when they marry, don't they? I used to play with dice as a kid, invent games around them. I took those dice into my first marriage, and I was kept entertained by my use of them as a cost-free harmless recreation. But I became a little bit embarrassed I was still 'using'. Sometimes I played dice on the sly when no-on was around. Was it an addiction? Whatever it was, it was surely better than alcohol or smoking. But I finally adhered to that biblical line that advises 'leave childish things behind'. Getting rid of my dice was akin to growing up. They went into the dustbin.

Giving them up was my way of crossing that great dividing line between child and adult.

Other adults, men and women, exposed to parenthood have had no chance to grow up themselves. They then can feel dispossessed of their youth, imprisoned by new responsibilities foisted upon them. Whatever alternative plans they may have had for their own lives have to be put aside. From then on marriage is all about economics, balancing the books and rearing children. It is no wonder love between two people can dissipate. A couple can soon lose sight of one another.

It is quite conceivable they may soon feel like strangers even unto themselves never able to explain who they have become or why they behave as they do. They may become disorientated and repeat behaviour that's not only distressing to themselves but to others. The inhabitants of a marriage are sometimes uncomfortable or unfulfilled in the place or ensuing situations. Maybe then they even resort to drugs or drink looking for fulfilment and then get further lost.

There's a lot to be recommended that a child receives the right kind of guidance and advice while growing up. Love is the best thing that can happen to a child growing up. It gives them the best chance in life. Receiving good and constructive advice and accepting that it comes from a caring source means that you're not left guessing which road to take at every crossroads you meet and reduces the prospect of you dropping down every conceivable pothole in the road.

I wasn't long past 18 years old having stayed on at school to pass my English 'A' level, which I was told emphatically by my teacher I had no chance of passing, that I married my girlfriend with us expecting our first child.

Writing this almost a lifetime away from those days, I can say it's a huge difference when you are finally free to be yourself and to make your own choices and to talk with anyone about anything as I am now able to do. Once I never felt I fitted in.

It took a long time for me to get here. And here's some advice, though it may bore family and friends around you if you do it, do talk to others to break any chains inside you feel may bind or repress you. Talk to anyone! Practise voicing your thoughts to search for the words that will reveal to others how confused you may be about your feelings or events around you. It is very necessary to voice how you feel and come to terms with why you feel the way you do. When you can vent in speech all those suppressed thoughts inside of you, when you're not scared of doing so, you finally have with words the tools for life, words at your disposal to understand things in a way that you never did before.

You may achieve this breakthrough by self-analysis or under your own steam, which is quite probably the most time-consuming route. The quickest way is likely by seeking the help of a therapist, the more expensive path. I might have achieved the same result sooner had I gone to a therapist, but I am stubborn. I'm like a tortoise who takes its time, but it gets there. I trusted in my own mind, my own ability to work things out and timing being everything, when to do it.

Whichever way you choose to do it, if you are reading this and struggling with identity, or with something deep inside of you that you can't right now find the words to communicate to others, you can and one day will get there if you try. You can finally free yourself and start being a truer version of yourself to others. You can start living your own life and it is never too late to start. Speak out and do it loudly if necessary. It takes guts, but you'll never know how strong you are until you face your demons.

CHAPTER ELEVEN

BREAKING INTO JOURNALISM

I could never have worked for the cancer charities without first having honed my journalistic skills and now I'll tell you how close I came to missing my first break into journalism. How many of us are persuaded by strange circumstance to believe there is such a thing as fate or destiny?

My journalistic career began on *the South Yorkshire Times*, but because of a remarkable circumstance it nearly did not. I was interviewed on the SYT, a newspaper with a 50,000-weekly circulation, by a proper gentleman editor named Sydney Hacking. I'd seen the likes of Sydney before portrayed on TV in the war films. He looked like an RAF officer during the Second World War. He was tall, tidy and with a trim moustache.

Mr Hacking was fortunate. He born in an age when his surname was not synonymous with a nefarious journalistic practice. Phone hacking long after he had passed gave journalists and journalism a bad name.

At the close of my one hour-long interview in his office in the then mining town of Mexborough I was offered the job of a junior reporter on the Sheffield edition of the *South Yorkshire Times*. The likeable athletic Sydney Hacking who played lawn tennis for Yorkshire, shook my hand warmly at the interview's conclusion and told me: "I think you will do well." I went away with those encouraging words ringing in my ears. I was happy. Other than being a pop star, journalism was the only other freedom road I could think of because I wasn't built for football which was another great escape from poverty or oblivion. When I played football in my youth, I avoided more of the brutal contact by playing on the wings and believing myself to be tricky, like the best of wingers are. When the headmaster of my secondary school decided to take the school 'upmarket' and switch to rugger from football I played on the wing there too. The headmaster switched the school game back to football again, after one humiliating defeat. None of us were rugby players. We were miraculously leading 6-0 at the interval against a private school but succumbed to a mountainous loss 76-6. Football was in our blood and rugger just wasn't.

Now back to Sydney Hacking.

Now Mr Hacking if you are out there as an electric current or as a collection of atoms or an angel looking down from another world, then yes I do think I did do well, as you predicted I would. I dedicate my path through journalism to you and to my English teacher the long, six feet plus and smiling Peter Price who once informed the whole class when I was 14. "We have a writer in our midst" – and he meant me. Thank you, gents, belatedly for preparing the way.

However, two weeks following my job interview I had not received the job confirmation from Mr Hacking who had told me emphatically that he would be in touch with me within days. I decided to contact the newspaper and ask to speak to the editor and gently nudge him. Was there any reason for the hold up, I would ask him?

I phoned and asked the receptionist to be transferred to the editor's office.

Seconds later a brusque voice answered the phone: "Ridyard," he said.

"I would like to speak to Mr Hacking, please" I asked politely.

"Mr Hacking is dead. I am the editor now."

"Oh dear," was the best I could utter. What do you say at a moment like that? Surely, it rarely happens. I broke a pregnant pause in the conversation during which I took time to consider this dramatic development before explaining: "I was interviewed by Mr Hacking a few weeks ago and he gave me a job."

"Oh it's you, is it?" Ridyard said, in a tone not especially pleased to hear from me.

This Ridyard fellow wasn't blaming me for what had happened was he? Mr Hacking hadn't been murdered, had he? The police hadn't circulated a photo fit with me as the prime suspect, had they?

"Yes, it's me," I replied, it almost sounding as if I was giving myself up for a crime.

"Mr Hacking died later the same day that he interviewed you. Fortunately for you the last thing he did was to pass confirmation of your appointment to his secretary."

Fortunate I was. Very.

Never was I more grateful that Mr Hacking had not only been a gentleman but also a man of ultra-efficiency to have done what he did only hours before he died.

I was particularly grateful because if I had been interviewed by the new editor Ridyard, I may never have got my first break into journalism. You can tell these things, you know! Ridyard and I scraped along. He didn't have much to do with me. Of course, I wasn't one of his protégés.

The *South Yorkshire Times* was a good grounding place for journalism – ask Michael Parkinson. Yes, that Michael Parkinson who interviewed every global star male and female, including mercurial boxer Mohammed Ali when he had his own Saturday evening prime spot The Parkinson talk show.

I was to learn that the deputy editor while I was there, a Mr John Broxholme had summoned Parky to his office to tear a strip off him for some misdemeanour and made a prediction he probably regretted but went into folklore: "You'll never make it in journalism," he told Parky.

It was rather like Decca Records later dying of embarrassment for telling The Beatles they'd never make it.

I must tell you about my earliest story on the South Yorkshire Times. I was responsible for a death. You carry that load with you through life as a journalist.

A woman called to give me the name of a friend of hers, an elderly woman who she said had the oldest living budgerigar in the country.

I telephoned this budgie owner and asked her: "Could we please do a story about you and your budgie. It's apparently the oldest in the country, and maybe it could be, quite possibly the oldest in the world".

"No," she said: "I wouldn't like the attention, and neither would he."

"If we did a story your budgie could make history. It would certainly feature in the Guinness Book of Records. The story may also encourage other budgie owners to treat and feed their birds a little better if you tell our readers the secrets of your bird's longevity."

"No," she repeated: "I don't think so."

Other budgie owners could learn from you then do their very best for their birds and then other birds might outlive your budgie. Think of the good you'll be doing for the whole budgie population."

I just kept on and on with this kind of psychobabble until she finally relented. She eventually agreed to allow her bird to be photographed. Our cockney photographer Harry went out to take its picture. He came back later that day.

"No story," he told me.

"What do you mean no story?" I quizzed.

"I mean the budgie is dead."

"Dead?"

"The flash from my camera killed it."

CHAPTER TWELVE

FITNESS RUNNING EVERYWHERE

There is little doubt that keeping fit does give you an advantage when later in life you face serious illness or cancer as I have. Fitness and I started a fling that began with cross country runs before lunch as a teenager at school, the fling ended up as a big love affair. Some of my teenage peers at school made life defining choices too by making the effort to go out on the cross-country course at lunchtime. They put on their shorts and singlets and vanished into the woods to secretly smoke their fags. Some of them smoke for a lifetime and no doubt a few may have caught cancer as a result.

In my lifetime I must have run around the world dozens of times if I'd counted the miles.

Because for a long time I refused to take a driving test and buy a car I was running everywhere. I was the fittest young man living in the steel town of Rotherham and I became the fastest young man of my age in the entire country when I went under 2 hrs 30 minutes for a marathon, and I appeared in Athletics Weekly as a result.

When I produced the best of my running efforts, I was training around 100 miles a week in preparation, a figure which defies belief to me now. Runners of that era were copying the exploits of a chap called David Bedford who did prodigious amounts of training and had broken through to star at 10,000 metres on the track. A role model to me, he was.

About Rotherham itself. Tommy Docherty who had managed Manchester United saw his reputation plummet by having an affair with a colleague's wife and he was sacked by that glamorous and rich club. It must have been the strangest penance for Tommy to have then gone on to manage minnows Rotherham United. I used to see Tommy in the flesh on Sundays because we went to the same church.

There wasn't much clean air in this mucky South Yorkshire town. To save money, I ran down the Sheffield Road there and back daily between Rotherham and Sheffield to attend work at The Sheffield Star. I used to run through air that was horribly orange tinged caused by the oxide discharges from the steelmaking factories. Tommy famously and cleverly remarked: "Rotherham is the only place where pigeons fly backwards."

I used to make sure I didn't breathe in too deeply when I ran past the steelworks so as not to destroy my lungs. Whether that did any good, I'll never know. I've breathed a lot of clean seaside air since to make up for it.

It wasn't until my late 30's that I bit the bullet and took my driving test in Walkley, Sheffield, where I had just bought a house. The city of Sheffield is built on so many hills it rivals Rome which also has seven.

Sebastian Coe the eventual Olympic 1500 metres champion used to run past my house at Walkley on his training sessions and striding those giant lumpy hills led him to fame, glory and fortune. Walkley has staggeringly steep hills for athletes to train on and it was no wonder the area bred so many formidable long-distance runners. It wasn't an area where you'd advise heavy smokers to live. Even walking those hills every day in Walkley might have brought on heart attacks.

I used to train on those hills too, but one of those hills was memorable particularly on a day when I was instructed to do a hill stop on my driving test.

I was told by an examiner to brake and hold the car steady with my feet prepared to balance between clutch, brake and accelerator pedals. So steep was the incline I felt in charge of a rocket stood vertical and ready to launch into the blue yonder. Instead of the car going upwards, or should I say forwards when I released the brake, I feared the car, a Mini, would retreat backwards at pace as soon as the traffic lights signalled green for go. It felt like any second that car with my feet trembling uncertainly on the foot controls, might topple backwards causing a major accident.

As this cancer thing nearly ended my life too quickly to write this, please remember it's written as if I'm in a church confessional booth purging myself of sin. Here is my confession. I am sure I was over the alcohol limit when I took my driving test. I cannot not have been.

I must have reeked of alcohol.

The previous night to my driving test, instead of sensibly getting an early night my girlfriend and I had an argument that lasted well past 4am – and my test was scheduled for 10am that day. By 10am I hadn't slept at all. The argument had festered because we were both drinking. Next morning, I met a photographer friend in the pub that was just around the corner from the test centre in Walkley. I told my mate Ernest what had happened: "I'm not sure I'm in a fit state to take the test, Ernest. I've had quite a night. Maybe I'm tired and over emotional. Maybe you could take it for me?" I suggested, only half kidding.

"You've jogged here, haven't you?" he said.

I had.

"Yes, but I jog everywhere, but I've been drinking throughout the night and into the early morning. Drinking seriously into the early morning."

Ernest was a man with a solution for everything and it nearly always involved alcohol and mints.

"I'll tell you what. I'll get you a half of lager from the bar. Have yourself the hair of the dog and see how you feel after that."

That's what friends are for.

As I left the pub to go to the test centre he passed me a mouthful of Polo mints, so that my breath was fresh, or at least minty, when I breathed upon the examiner.

And so it was that I took my driving test – and somewhat miraculously I passed it.

When the car was stationary. much to my relief, after my drive, the invigilator handed me a document.

"I'm pleased to be able to tell you that you have passed your driving test, Mr Charnley, please sign this form."

With great difficulty I took the pen she offered me, and my hand shook like a leaf. I promise you it has never shaken as furiously since.

"Well, Mr Charnley, in all the tests I have taken I have never met anyone quite as nervous as you are," she observed.

I went back to the pub to give Ernest the good news and we celebrated my success with a few more beers.

In my chosen profession, journalism, you had to sign indentures which meant you were tied to your first newspaper for three and half years on slave wages. I used to run everywhere to cover my reporting jobs and I wouldn't have survived financially had I not. Yes, I ran everywhere in all weathers and sharpish.

I couldn't afford a car, hadn't then passed a driving test and anyway I was a keen and stringy long-distance runner. I ran my first marathon under-age at 18. A friend of mine recently reminded me of that race. He ran it alongside me he recalled. He was a novice too. It was in held in Rotherham, the Rotherham Harriers Marathon. In those days they had no water stations along the route. I ran in well-worn canvas shoes more like pumps and more notably I ran in temperatures that day that rose above 85 degrees. It was a marathon baptism of fire.

It's etched in my memory because I remember reaching a point where I was totally disorientated at around 20 miles, some runners refer to it these days as 'hitting the wall'. You feel you can go no further. In deadly heat on the baking streets, I realised I was no longer running in a straight line. This was pointed out to me by a pedestrian standing at the roadside.

"Oy. You're going around in circles, mate."

I had started to run in ever decreasing circles in the road in an exhausted state badly needing rehydrating. My head had been fried by the sun. My running buddy Brian Mullarkey recalled that his mother saved the day for both of us by rushing to a shop and buying us each an ice lolly. How on earth I still finished in around 3 hours 20 minutes I shall never know. Better marathon times were to come.

My newspaper indentures completed after sitting in on enough boring parish council meetings to last me a lifetime, I took my journalism proficiency test. This tested my knowledge of law, government and the rest, but the most difficult part of the examination was shorthand. Reporters always swore by a method called Pitman's but learning that would have defeated me. It was too complex. As it was, thankfully someone had just come up with another shorthand which was easier called Teeline and thanks to that I managed the minimum 100 words a minute that would allow me to cover almost anything necessary word for word reporting in the magistrates and crown courts.

Incidentally, it used to amuse me in the courts when police officers gave their evidence in twos and obviously lied each and every time they appeared in the witness box. They did so but nobody challenged them and that included me.

The chief magistrate would ask two policemen separately when they had made up their notes of a particular incident asking if there had been any collusion when their notes were made? Were they made independently and away from each other? No collusion, they always replied.

But every two officers presenting their evidence in court quoting from their notebooks had written down identical accounts, every word the same, every full stop and comma the same as their colleagues. Yet they swore in court they had achieved this while apart and written at different times. Either most South Yorkshire Policemen lied, or they were clairvoyant with one other.

I went from the *South Yorkshire Times* for an interview at *The Sheffield Star*. It's circulation then was over 100,000 copies a night. It was a big deal to get onto this newspaper.

I was told there were more than 100 applicants for three reporting vacancies.

In those days, unlike today, newspapers were highly successful and hugely influential, and the Sheffield Star was one of the biggest and best publications in the country. It paid well too.

There were more journalists in employment in this country in my day than you can ever imagine but the competition to work on these monoliths was intense. Graduates speaking with posh voices, plenty of them with trim beards, filled most of the seats in newsrooms on all provincial evening newspapers.

I was interviewed by a guy I liked called Peter Goodman, who was the deputy editor of *The Star* and a guy who was a little more challenging called David Mastin, and he was the news editor. I thought at the time they were playing Mr Nice and Mr Nasty as they did on police fiction shows on TV.

One policeman had to be so nasty that the criminal would confess to the nice policeman who would be befriending him. They fooled the criminal by acting in that way and always got to the truth. Mastin I thought was being unreasonably dour and combative whenever I answered a question.

It would have been some comfort to both that neither died shortly after my interview as did Mr Hacking when he gave me my first reporting job. Had these two been told about my only previous newspaper interview they might have cancelled mine with The Star thinking it was the kiss of death for them. Had either of them died I may have been forced to consider visiting a priest capable of performing an exorcism on me.

Anyway, having survived Mr Nasty's taunts and his unsmiling demeanour I was taken on and he became my unsmiling, taunting news editor whose catchphrase to his reporters – or was it just me – was 'keep smiling'. It was a big bump up on wages for me and there must have been more than 150 reporters on the floor of Sheffield Newspapers office working for its two titles *The Star* and *The Morning Telegraph*.

Now as an eleven plus school failure, journalism should not have been a career option for the likes of me. Eleven plus failures, who were my school peers of this time ended up working in shops or on the buses driving or conducting. But most the lads ended up down the coal mine or in the steel works and it was thanks to the unions they could earn themselves decent money. Instead, I found myself working alongside graduates from universities all over the country including Oxbridge.

There was a rich history of individuals who had worked on The Star and made a name for themselves. One was Len Doherty who had been a miner but, like me had a poor school background, being schooled in the same mining area as myself. He still made it onto this top regional newspaper. His was an inspiring story. You do need your role models. Doherty later made his name also by facing up to terrorist hijackers on a plane. Sadly, Len's story ended badly. He took his own life.

On the brighter side I was once having a lunchtime beer in a pub with another journalist, a likeable public school educated cockney called Max learning his trade on The Star and told him I had ambition to get my music heard by a wider audience. He replied: "Well they laughed at one journalist who worked here in the Rotherham office of *The Sheffield Star*. He said he was going to write books…"

"And did he? Who was it they laughed at?" I asked.

It turned out that this aspiring book writer, this local journalist, was David Nobbs and he went on to become one very successful writer spurning one of TV's great characters Reginald Perrin, played by Leonard Rossiter. '*The Rise and Fall of Reginald Perrin*'.

I thought his first book called '*Pratt of The Argus*' was hilarious and very close to home. Nobbs wrote comedic fiction, and his earliest work was based on his reporting life in South Yorkshire. He didn't either bother disguising many of the names or characters who appeared in his early work. They were people he worked with, as I did later.

It was while working on *The Sheffield Star* that I accidentally got closer to Her Majesty Queen Elizabeth than I should have.

I was scheduled to cover The Queen's official opening of the Herringthorpe Leisure Centre in Rotherham and the previous night I had been on stage singing with my band. After we got home to my place after the gig many of the band stayed around drinking at my house and we forgot about time.

I was due to be at the leisure centre at around 9am next morning and the next thing I knew when I checked the time there was about half an hour left to get to my royal appointment. It was panic stations. I called a taxi and it sped me there.

I told the taxi driver to get as close to the centre as he could. By now crowds were massing and noisily waiting to see more of their royal guest who had now gone inside.

I was now officially late and instructed the taxi driver to get ever closer.

"Here, I'll get out here," I said, and he stopped his vehicle with a crowd now gathering around us. I think they wanted to see which of the royal family was arriving late in a Rotherham taxi.

I didn't realise I'd urged the driver on to such an extent that when I got out, I didn't have far to hoof it on foot before I was walking on a red carpet.

What I had failed to do when I got home from my gig the previous night was to change out of my stage gear.

At the leisure centre I was wearing an all-white suit with my long dyed red burnt hair flowing down my back and I hobbled on white platform shoes. My God, I must have looked like a royal or Gary Glitter, who then wasn't disgraced as in later years he become.

It was a good job I did look like royalty because by continuing to walk the red carpet, it led m me directly to join the royal entourage and there I was stood just a few feet from the queen. I looked around in amazement and saw on the other side of the hall my fellow members of the press standing behind a roped off area. Knowing who I was, they were pointing fingers at me obviously wanting to ask one question: "How the bloody hell did you get there?"

The strange thing was I wasn't challenged at all and as the group meandered off. I followed, as regally as I could as part of this VIP group.

At one point I was fifth in line, not to the throne but with Her Majesty leading our select band along a second floor corridor.

Then we went out onto a balcony, just a select few of us. Not all braved the open air because not all could be accommodated, and I was one of the fortunate few looking down below on thousands of The Queen's subjects as she gave them graciously that all familiar wave of hers with me stood just behind her doing my bit by smiling for the crowd while trying to remain innocuous.

I can only think that council officials thought that looking as I did in my white suit, I was part of the royal family, a lesser-known royal, a mad uncle or nephew and the royal party would have been thinking I was one of the council officials who had dressed appropriately in order to accompany them

I was to be at close quarters with Queen Elizabeth again when I later worked on the *Windsor & Eton Express* and attended a church service at Christmas. There I was standing outside while a lone photographer took pictures of the royal group. I was again just feet away from the Queen. The photographer and I were on reporting duty in the unlikely event anything untoward happened at or after the ceremony. We would have alerted the press agency in the event of anything shocking.

Queen Elizabeth wouldn't have recognised me without my white platform shoes.

To any young people reading this, if you are told to listen to your career officer but they register with you immediately as a dolt, someone negative about your prospects and failing to pick-up on your burning ambition or talent then tell them as politely as they deserve to be told that they don't know what they are talking about and suggest they find themselves another job and get out of your face.

The careers officer who came to visit me at my school was unforgettable for all the wrong reasons. He informed me he had already met more than a dozen pupils at the Grammar School in my town, boys and girls who all desired to be journalists and told me they would go on to achieve higher qualifications than I would. He followed up by asking me my preference, was it to work down the coal mine or in the steelworks. If neither of those opportunities appealed, he said – though that was where the money was earned he reminded me – I could always work in a shop if I didn't mind working on Saturdays which meant he said I wouldn't be able to play football or support my local professional football team.

At school they even arranged trips to the mine and steelworks for us lads so we could see what the future held in store for us.

I remember a trip into the steelworks between Rotherham and Sheffield – the one I used to run past daily through an orange mist when I became a journalist – as if it was yesterday. It was like entering the fires of hell.

Men some bare chested stood before massive flames and there were continuous and incredibly loud sounds of metal being struck on metal. Men wore earmuffs and stood bronzed like statues watching the various head banging processes these repeated day on day on day. These men earned their money and deserved more for bearing the grim working conditions the perpetual noise and stifling heat. As for the mines, from time to time there were always mining disasters underground where men lost their lives.

Later as a reporter covering inquests many of the deaths of ageing miners were from pneumoconiosis, the common lung disease caught by miners' underground. I couldn't help but feel that I had dodged a bullet not going underground.

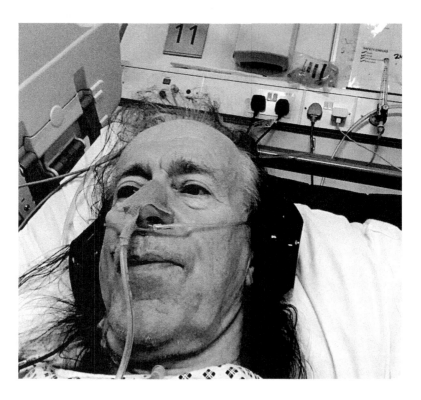

Alan post operational

CHAPTER THIRTEEN

MORE PRE-OPERATIVE ADVICE
FOR SCAREDY CATS

Returning from my relevant and necessary leap into the past from Nagasaki, Japan and the effects of the atom bomb, from my tales of a distant mother, of my work beginnings and here I am now with more advice for my fellow scaredy cats – so listen in.

I had been diagnosed with cancer. You can't choose what life throws at you, but you can control how you deal with it.

A word of warning to anyone facing a string of hospital appointments that may seem endless. While visiting hospital you will be relentlessly checked as to your identity repeatedly. I have never parroted my name, birthdate and first line of my address and postal code so often. At times I likened myself to a Second World War prisoner who after arrest by the enemy was required by his regiment even under duress to reveal only his serial number.

If you're in the hospital system you may also be required to wear a wrist tag that they'll have ready made for you, giving you a bonus of knowing who you are in the unlikely event that you become confused and forget!

But because of these identity precautions you can be certain too that you will not be mistaken for another patient and have a whole leg removed instead of a small lump.

Pre-operation, I never truly saw my surgeon without a mask because my treatment occurred during the Covid outbreak and yes because covid was rampant I underwent plenty of those, to me, horrible covid tests. Who enjoys retching when a stick is put down your throat? I had been isolating at home with my good lady Gillian during Covid as she was particularly vulnerable. A great fear at the time during what was a pandemic was the threat of catching serious covid symptoms that led to breathing problems. That could eventually lead to hospitalisation and in the worst circumstance being placed on a ventilator to be kept alive.

These were grim times. Deaths from covid in hospital convinced just about everyone to think that hospital was a dangerous place to go even if you felt extremely unwell. An appointment was to be avoided at all costs. Visitors were forbidden permission to visit loved ones. You could be admitted into hospital with one complaint and catch another, Covid, despite the hospital's best efforts.

Many who were admitted with Covid or caught it in there never came out. But many people in desperate need of treatment didn't go for help when perhaps they should have. I decided to chance it.

In 2022, thanks to Covid there was a staggering backlog of cancer patients waiting longer for treatment with longer waiting times.

Now my surgeon's height and his features that I could make out beyond the covid mask reminded me of someone else and who that was I couldn't quite fathom. I later realised he had a similarity in looks to Martin Clunes who played the popular TV role of *Doc Martin*, the doc handicapped because he couldn't stand the sight of blood.

My consultant surgeon must have been nothing like Doc Martin. He must have seen gallons of my blood during an eight-hour operation because I needed a blood transfusion as this beast of a tumour of mine from my bowel plus one more, a tumour in my prostate, were removed. I had signed my tumour over to the hospital's research centre. I hoped one day it wouldn't grow legs, escape from a laboratory, and track me down.

I watch too much sci-fi. Is there a chance too I could become a film star because of my treatment? You see I also signed a form that allowed them to film my operation.

"Don't worry they won't know it's you and they won't show your face," said the nurse advising me about their filming procedure beforehand – ever the showman – I signed.

I signed on the line recognising that I would become only as famous as say the actor who played '*The Invisible Man*'.

My satisfaction was to be that trainee surgeons could watch the two experts operating on me and admire and copy their expertise. Once again looking for positives about the outcome of my operation, surely the surgeons being filmed operating on me would be out to make an impression. The last thing they'd want to do would be to cock up my operation and have their film released under the title '*How Not to Operate on a Patient*'.

Of course, before going under general anaesthetic, as a patient you should make sure you are not worrying unnecessarily about incredible one-off and bizarre incidents you may have heard others speak gravely about before, like what goes wrong on the operating table?

Some of these stories are nothing more than old wives' tales or bad folklore, probably concerning the one in a million operation that does go crazily wrong. I refer to a surgeon leaving a scalpel or some other surgical tool inside of you.

You have as much chance of that occurring as you have of scooping the top prize in the National Lottery. I recall reading one story too about a man who walked off the street and who posing as a surgeon performed operations when unqualified. Now how likely is that to happen? Mind you, with everyone wearing Covid masks these days a doctor in an operating theatre might have no idea of the qualifications or identity of the man or woman standing next to him…. gulp.

Another worry more common than it should be, and you may have read patients accounts of this in popular women's magazines is the '*I was wide awake as they operated on me*' account. That's a nightmare scenario too but with scant chance of it occurring.

"I couldn't move, and I wanted to scream for them to stop the operation, but I couldn't, and I felt the pain of very second of the procedure…" the woman in the article in a popular women's magazine will be quoted as saying, pooh-poohing the anaesthetist whose expert advice was that it rarely if ever happened – and the storyteller getting paid enormous amounts of money into her account for telling lies. She may be just an attention or money seeker or just a plain old liar.

Pay no heed to this type of story.

From my experience under general anaesthetic, you are unconscious. I don't remember any dreaming when I was out cold. I certainly didn't have a nightmare as I did as a boy with Mr Dread the Dentist and his gas.

With the general anaesthetic, as I've mentioned, it is no time before the needle goes in and then you blackout and then your eyes open and you have no memory of anything that happened to you in between time Perfect.

You are unconscious then wake to find your operation over. That being the case, why waste time worrying about your operation unnecessarily, after all the odds are with you. It seldom goes wrong. Have trust.

At pre-op sessions they are required to furnish you with statistics about the risk to your life during a particular operation.

Once at my meeting with my surgeon it was put at between 0.6 per cent and two per cent and the highest estimate of a demise was when I spoke to a pre-op anaesthetist who warned "the risk with some was in certain circumstances up to 10 per cent but I wouldn't even think about that in your case," he advised with a knowing smile.

That high percentage of low-rate survival appertained to people with pre-existing conditions or maybe gross obesity, which doesn't help your cause.

Before my appointment with the anaesthetist, I was told every pre-op candidate had to do a fitness test on an exercise bike. This was to measure breathing and cardiac responses.

I was looking forward to this. If there was a record to beat for riding this stationary bike in that man's office and an Olympic cyclist hadn't been aboard it already, then I wanted a crack at it. It sounded like fun. But when the anaesthetist read my fitness notes he told me: "No, we don't need to bother with the bike in your case." I was exasperated, frustrated, disappointed, like a boy who'd just had a toy snatched away. Good job they didn't take my blood pressure when he refused me my bike ride!

About fitness.

Before the operation if you or the doctors consider you less fit than perhaps you should be before an operation, there's usually a window of opportunity beforehand to improve fitness and breathing by doing things you may have avoided before – like walking to the shop a few times instead of hopping into your car. Tackling a few press ups. Joining a gym to do some gentle jerks.

Nothing excessive, of course.

Fitness does help you through ops. It doesn't though help you if you carry excessive weight into the operating theatre.

I had reconciled myself to the actual tumour removal operation under general anaesthetic, but the anaesthetist then added an unwanted surprise. You will always get one or two of these surprises. You must take them in your stride: "I advise you to have an epidural," he said.

Oh dear.

"It will make things easier for you after the operation. You can be fed intravenously afterwards, for instance."

How many women have had epidurals while undergoing caesarean births and not batted an eyelid? I'd heard that the needle into the spine was painful. But the injection would only take less than a minute. Just do it, I told myself. It's never as bad as it's been made out to be and it's over in a jiffy my inner sense was spouting to me: "Okay I told him an epidural it is," though of course I didn't relish that prospect.

As I left the room the anaesthetist surprised me by saying: "You're the best patient I've had in weeks."

I had listened to an expert and not voiced fears and agreed with a someone who knew his onions.

That anaesthetist along with my surgeon would make up the team that was being assembled to accompany me on my rocket trip to the moon. I was going to be in good hands. Why worry?

As part of my post-operative care, I was duly connected by tube to be drip fed, By the time they had finished with me I also had surgical drains that are implants.

Surgical drains are tubes placed near surgical incisions in the post-operative patient, to remove pus, blood or other fluid, preventing it from accumulating in the body.

The type of drainage system inserted is based on the needs of patient, type of surgery, type of wound, amount of drainage expected and surgeon preference.

These allow removal of fluid or gas from a wound or body cavity. I also had stents in the area of the stoma.

You know none of these insertions have happened until you wake up and gingerly try moving. This is where having some experience of bondage comes in handy! Struggle is useless. Relax and let the healing process begin.

Stents and drains are removed painlessly by nurses usually just before you leave the hospital for home. They are so good to get rid of. You have your body back.

CHAPTER FOURTEEN

MEN IN TIGHTS & SINGING IN THE WARD

Men in tights – the future of gender fluid fashion? It's already happening big time in our hospitals…

Film maker Mel Brooks was there first promoting this kind of leg wear in his film *'Robin Hood-Men in Tights'*.

But men of a certain age or persuasion would still balk at slipping on a pair. If you're a man in hospital for major surgery you'd better get used to being measured up for a pair to wear – and trust me, they'll be the tightest of tights you will ever be squeezed into. Even you women, who will wear them too will find them exceedingly tight if not strangulating.

Incidentally mine were white. Maybe they all are in hospital. They didn't ask me if I had a colour preference.

It was a surprise to me when a nurse arrived in pre-op and said she had to fit me up with a pair. I asked myself a question. Was I going to star in the hospital pantomime? Out she took a tape measure to establish my inside leg measurement.

Pulling on the tightest of tights are what all blokes are required to do as well as the women in hospitals, when they go for certain operations.

133

Tights are worn so that a blood clot doesn't travel up your legs and then onwards into your blood stream causing something nasty to happen to you while you're flat out on the operating table.

You will wear them for a while afterwards too and you are also given injections of blood thinners in your tummy or thigh. Self-injection at home was necessary for four weeks after I left hospital – and I was still wearing those tights for a few weeks at home as instructed although my sharp toenails eventually burst through the feet of each pair, the beginning of the end of all pairs I possessed.

I'm told people wear these tights on aeroplanes to prevent embolisms. You pull them up high to your thighs. Good job they don't go any higher or they could strangle you.

One nurse while I was in hospital helped me on with a pair after the operation, because they are exceedingly difficult to pull up. We were both tugging in the same direction when she noticed something about my legs…

"Do you know, you have exactly the same shaped legs as me," she remarked as she gazed down at my now tightly covered pins.

Is there an answer to that? If there is I didn't produce it at the time. Yes, we both had two legs, but surely there any comparison faltered or ended?

I remember being woozy under medication at the time so as the nurse left my ward cubicle, I failed to study her legs as she left. I will regret not doing so for the rest of my life. I am hoping and suspecting that she did have rather nice legs. Incidentally my own legs are thin as a rake through a lifetime of walking and running that's probably why mine resembled hers.

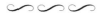

I sang to my fellow patients on Ward 10 at the Christie cancer Hospital Manchester one morning just a few days after my major operation to remove one tumour – they found a second one too and extricated that from my prostate.

Most men get prostate cancer but don't die of it unless it is particularly aggressive. Mine was an angry one, I was assured. My operation was one for the price of two tumours. Not a bad result and post operation they told me they had also removed my appendix, a useless body organ I am informed.

Anyway, there were kind compliments about my serenading post-operation in the hospital ward that morning. I must have been full of the joys of spring knowing my body invaders had been eliminated. One of the patients with not such a good diagnosis beamed to me a radiant smile and remarked about my singing of songs: "That has really raised my spirits," he said.

Okay you devil's advocates, not trusting a word I write. You may suggest that fellow patients had no choice but to listen as they were bedbound confined and restricted by their operation wounds.

I was making suffering patients endure more pain and they couldn't get at me to silence me, the poor souls.

The worst amongst you doubters of my singing ability may suggest too those hearing me were grimacing and not smiling.

You will allege I was being paid by the NHS to carry out a secret ambush on these patients to punish them for costing the service so much money. You may argue these patients were reluctant to attempt escape from my warbling less they over-extended themselves and burst their stitches.

Yes, I might have used all of these suggestions as to what might happen as an excuse not to sing. It's easy to put yourself off doing something that is positive.

Always think positive. Just do what needs to be done or what you feel should. Actions speak louder than words.

Doctors and nurses went by on the corridor adjoining the ward as I sang the Bill Withers *'Lovely Day'* and the Frankie Valli's *'Can't Take My Eyes Off You'*, amongst other golden oldies. I received overall thumbs up and smiles aplenty from these passers-by too, though okay, that last assertion about the smiles was guesswork because I was reduced to seeing only their expressive smiling eyes of approval because the joy was hidden behind covid masks. I could tell by their body language they were enjoying it. I'm sure too I drew dance steps from one or two.

Music is a great cheerer upper and means so much to a great many people. I was careful not to play any of my original sad songs, the type I had written from childhood. There would be no tears that day, no breaking of hearts or slashing of wrists.

I had brought my covers show backing tracks into the hospital on an I-pad. I sang naturally without a microphone. I've always loved singing.

I'd now like to go and sing to the sick especially at the local hospice as soon as my recovery is complete – I'm six weeks into that recovery at present and they say it can take three to six months to recover completely. Some people I'm told take a year. As my body starts the process of repairing itself, I'm already starting to feel good and buoyant, with only the occasional blip. As I write this, I'm in my fourth week of not driving.

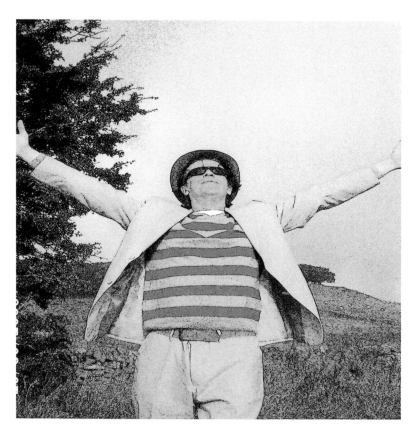

Alan in latest guise as Johnny Dysfunctional

CHAPTER FIFTEEN

SIGNED BY A MAJOR RECORD LABEL

I told you I sang on the cancer ward at The Christie Hospital after my major operation to remove two tumours.

I have sung all my life but never had I sang in a hospital nor after a major operation!

These days I go by the name of Johnny Dysfunctional and here's a link to some songs.

When Covid struck the only advice that the Government had for us was to wash our hands. This made a great song. What else but '*Wash Your Hands*'. I enlisted actors from all over the world to wash their hands and dance in a unifying gesture. Have a look and listen,

https://www.youtube.com/watch?v=4En3XpAtwNw

Wash Your Hands Beat the Virus Johnny Dysfunctional – YouTube

Further back in my history, and while working for *The Star* at its Rotherham office I got signed by CBS Records in my early 20's. They also gave me a publishing contract with April Music. My first record was to be released on the Epic label, the same label as ABBA were on.

When I presented my recording contract, a weighty document, for a lawyer in Rotherham to look over he hadn't seen the likes of one before. There were no music business lawyers in Rotherham because no-one in the down-at-heel town ever won a deal from a major record label. Music lawyers setting up shop in Rotherham would have starved. Most musicians did too.

My lawyer might have been reading the contract upside down for all the sense it made to him. In general terms it enslaved me to CBS, however in exchange I'd have fortune and fame. Which hungry young boy doesn't sign on the line with undue haste? But before CBS and this contract there had been plenty of 'pop' world experience preliminaries coming my way.

My music adventure started when at school I was in bands. I'd do paid work as the singer two or three nights a week at smoke filled packed pubs and working men's clubs. It's worth mentioning here that all round TV star and entertainer and trumpeter Roy Castle played those clubs and though he didn't smoke himself he died from cancer, thought to have been caused by inhaling smoke while trumpeting.

One of my claims to fame is that on two separate occasions in large sized clubs, punters who were listening to my singing came into my dressing room after my performances and told me that their drinking glasses in front of them had shattered when I had hit high notes. Make of that what you will. I could really hit those high falsetto notes...

The band with whom I was singing was good and we auditioned at London's legendary Tin Pan Alley for a lengthy summer residency abroad. We passed that audition.

Our suitcases were packed, and we were in our agent's office in Yorkshire ready to travel to a warmer climate when he took a phone call. We couldn't go. Couldn't get the insurance for us. Our residency was at the Cat's Eyes Club in Beirut. War had just broken out in Beirut. You may ask, when isn't there war in Beirut? It was one of those life changing moments. The Beatles learned their trade in Hamburg. If we could have handled bombs dropping around us during our performances in Beirut, nothing would have stopped us hitting the top.

I explained to you that I wrote music from an early stage of my life as a way of expressing denied feelings. Well, it turned out that people in the music business sniffed that I had a special talent. One of the highlights of working for CBS was walking into a studio in Whitfield Street to record a vocal and hearing a full orchestra playing two of the songs I had written in my bedroom.

In my raw naivety and possibly indicating to others that I had just landed from a backward planet, later during that very same day at the studio I was clandestinely interviewing some of the session musicians CBS had lined up to play on my music. I was thinking in terms of recruiting them. The keyboard player, for instance. He was very good. I'd maybe interest him too after all he was already playing my material!

"Hi, are you doing much these days? Fancy joining a (My) band?"

It was a musician called Alan Hawkshaw.

I didn't know he'd been doing bits and bobs with *David Bowie* and was in *The Shadows* for a time, but that proved at least I was a good judge of talent. I'd have paid him in buttons and dreams.

Later Hawkshaw wrote the *Grange Hill* TV series theme tune as well as The *Countdown* Theme which played every night for donkey's years on Channel 4 and is still being played. It must have earned its writer a fortune.

Also playing on my session that day was bass player Les Hurdle who'd played with Lou Reed and Donna Summer and who also became a Womble with Mike Batt and there was also Frank Ricotti the jazz vibraphonist and percussionist who has played on nearly everybody's sessions but including Freddie Mercury and The Pet Shop Boys. I also got the Mike Mansfield Orchestra on that day.

But there had been other suitors recognising my talent before CBS signed me. While on *The Star* in Sheffield I wrote a story about the writer of the TV series Z Cars theme, John Keating running a contest to find a song that the fans of Sheffield United could sing on the terraces. I thought that while I was writing that story I might as well enter the song contest too and I did. I came runner up too, even though at the time Rotherham United and not Sheffield United was my favourite South Yorkshire club.

There was another situation that occurred rather like that later in my reporting life and its worth relating.

While working on the Bournemouth Evening as a sports sub editor I had to stay behind and do a late afternoon shift placing the horse racing results in the stop press column. It meant hanging around the office doing nothing but awaiting those York results. For a bit of excitement, I nipped to the betting office and picked six horses in the Ebor race meeting at York.

As the horse racing results came into the newspaper office in dribs and drabs from York, so my disbelief grew. I had picked two winners at around 6-1, one at 16-1 and another at very long odds.

By the time it came to the last race I needed a horse called Sir Joey to win and then – I was informed later – I would have won £72,000! Sir Joey let me down and it started the race at odds of 28-1 but I still picked up just over £3,000. Sir Joey stormed to victory in his next race appearance just to make me feel sick.

However, that song success with the Z Cars man writing the Sheffield United song came at a cruel price. That infernal; melody and lyric became an earworm that I have never been able to shake. The chorus lyric expresses: '*And you know Sheffield United hate to lose, hate to lose, yes you know Sheffield United hate to lose*'. It still plays stubbornly on and on and on in my head.

I was 'discovered' a second time, after my Keating effort, by one of the Beachboys, the writer of *Disney Girls*, Bruce Johnston. Bruce had formed a partnership with a guy called Terry Melcher and they were starting a new record label.

I had sent off a tape to him – all the way to America. It was a miracle I'd been able to afford the postage.

I believe in this 'we are all separated by just three degrees' spookiness. But try the seven levels of separation explanation first and you'll get the idea. That is, 'if you speak to enough people about enough people, someone is going to know someone who knows someone who ultimately knows you. No matter where you are in the world, we are only separated by seven levels This is how a humble guy on the breadline in Rotherham made a connection not only with a world-famous musician but also by proxy with the murderer and madman Charlie Manson.

You see, Melcher, who was Doris Day's son, rejected Charles Manson's talents as a musician in the USA. Manson was so annoyed by this decision he was to become the mastermind of a killing spree at Melcher's house. He mistakenly believed Melcher to be still living there. Melcher wasn't at the time. He had moved on. Melcher had let the house to the film producer Roman Polanski, and it was his pregnant girlfriend Sharon Tate who was manically stabbed to death by Manson's hippy disciples who were part of his cult.

That aside you arguably couldn't get much better a producer at that time than Melcher who was at the recording desk for the making of the Byrds singles *Mr Tambourine Man* and *Turn, Turn, Turn*.

I met the Beachboy Bruce Johnston to discuss being signed to his and Melcher's new US record label at a top floor spacious room at the Inn on the Park, the lush five-star London hotel, a room with an amazing shag pile carpet and a TV that rose from below floor level at the flick of a switch.

While I had beforehand waited in the foyer to meet Bruce, I noticed the place was brimming with oil rich Arabs wearing their impressive white robes and headscarves. But for the heavy rain outside, I could have been mooching around in a hotel in the Middle East.

Bruce was a trim blue stylishly suited and booted gentlemen and he said he had just concluded some business deal. He could have doubled as a banker that day. He was genial and polite. He said: "I sure love your song."

He was referring to Rainmaker.

As usual it was one of my sad songs. Boy leaves girl and regrets his silly actions that led to the break-up.

"Thank you," I replied.

"You shouldn't though try to sound like the Beach Boys. What you should do is find your own sound," he then said.

What?

"But we could do something with that song of yours."

Instead of saying 'great, what do you plan to do with Rainmaker' or 'how exciting it must be for you that you plan to run your own record label,' instead I took the wrong direction.

"I'm not trying to sound like the Beach Boys," I argued: "I am, sounding like myself." I was only being true to myself explaining this to Mr Johnston. Wouldn't a nice man like him appreciate my honesty?

I learned instead, it is inadvisable to start an argument with one of the world's most celebrated musicians in one of the world's biggest bands, even if you're being frank and honest.

"Well, who is your favourite band?" he asked.

That was a cue for me to have leapt back into his good books.

With hindsight my reply should obviously have been The Beach Boys. But that would have backed up his claim that I was trying to sound like his band, or even to write like him. I think he wanted me to back down and admit, "Okay, yes I am heavily influenced by the Beach Boys and by you especially. You were right."

If I had taken that route, then fortune and fame would then have followed with Terry Melcher, the Byrds record producer at the recording console.

However, there were absolutely no surfers in the coal and steel town of Rotherham where I'd just travelled down to the south from. On the jukeboxes in that town the Beachboys hardly figured. It was more than a hundred miles from there to the nearest surfer absent beach resort where the sun wouldn't be that hot either. The discs on the town's juke boxes offered mainly heavy rock. It was more of a Rolling Stone's or heavy metal town, just like it was a predictable town that voted every election time Labour and not Conservative and that was even if the Labour candidate was a sack of potatoes.

"My favourite band. It's '*The Association*'," I told Bruce.

Oh dear. Bad choice.

I think from that moment Bruce cooled on me. That band '*The Association*' I did not know then were bitter, bitter rivals of The Beachboys. They battled regularly over the top spot in the States charts with each single release.

I'd told Bruce the truth. I loved the harmonies of The Association above any band, even though I did think the Beach Boys were very special and '*God Only Knows*' is still one of my all-time favourite songs. Why didn't I just tell him that? And '*Wouldn't It Be Nice*' is great too. But among my all-time favourites too are The Association numbers '*Cherish*' '*Never My Love*' and '*Requiem to The Masses*'.

Bruce was very kind. He gave me a calling card. He said: "Look why don't you go along to Rocket Records and see my friend

Elton John. Tell him Bruce sent you. I'm sure he'll be interested in what you've got. I do love that song," I thanked him and left.

When I returned to Rotherham, in no time I carefully wrapped and despatched a tape to Elton's Rocket Records label and then having heard nothing back despite playing my ace card in a letter that Bruce Johnston of the world-famous Beachboys had asked me to get in touch with Elton, I then followed up with a visit to Rocket.

I got to see the man in charge that day. He wore a crumpled suit. His nose was running. He didn't stand to shake my hand when I offered it. He remained behind his desk. He looked worse for wear and flummoxed when I told him Bruce had sent me to see Elton personally.

"You sent a tape in?" he asked.

"Yes, a fortnight ago and I thought that as I hadn't heard from you, I'd follow it up quickly with a visit."

"Just a moment," he said and unsteadily stood up.

He made his way over to the corner of a room where stood what looked to be a giant waste-paper container. It was over-flowing with tapes.

"What does your tape look like?" he asked.

I couldn't think of any distinguishing marks. I wished now I'd wrapped it in pink paper with a purple ribbon.

He waded in with both arms. He was splashing out, next to swimming in his waste bin of discarded tapes. There must have been hundreds in there, probably all unheard and he was prob-ably off his head.

My guess had been that it wasn't a summer cold that made his nose run it was coke sniffing. He didn't even have a clue what he was looking for in the waste bin. It was quite some filing system he had organised. I had no patience with him. I was so disgusted I left. "Never mind," I said. That is how I never met Elton John yet had been supposed to!

The A & R man who signed me for CBS Records was Lem Lubin, a nice fellow who told me he had perfect pitch and he'd had a big hit in a band called Unit 4 Plus 2 with '*Concrete and Clay*'. *He* told me: "Being signed by CBS is like winning the lottery."

Lem later had a big hit after transferring from CBS to Elton's Rocket Records with Judy Tsuke and a dreamy song called '*Stay With Me Till Dawn*'. If I'd hung around he could have taken me with him to Elton's label.

After I had unceremoniously left CBS, I got a nice message from Lem posted to my home address: 'Keep the faith,' it said.

Another nice guy who called me after CBS dramatically changed its musical taste from me to *The Clash* was Tony Rivers. Tony and his team had sung all the harmonies on my songs at CBS studios – and they were top class. Tony and his crew were on so many hit records of the time and one of their finest moments was on '*Miss You Nights*' by Cliff Richard. Give it a listen and you'll see what I mean. They sang great on two of my songs.

Was being signed by CBS like winning the lottery? I didn't think so at the time. I thought I was there on merit. I write good songs and still do. I believed totally that it was my calling.

I had always listened to and loved music, one of my earliest memories was as a newly married young man hearing for the first time Glen Campbell singing a Jimmy Webb composition called *'Wichita Lineman'*. The day I heard that song in the bathroom on my tinny transistor radio I was transported to a snow torn scene somewhere in America where a lone and lonely lineman was working on restoring a telephone line and while doing so was listening in on the lines to others' conversations. Magic.

My first single release for CBS was that song Beachboy Bruce favoured called *'Rainmaker'*. Yes, you remember, the sad song about the break-up of a romance. I had recorded a demo on which I sang played bass and keyboards at a place called Fairview Studios at Hull and it sounded just great.

Fairview had become a mecca for Northern rock outfit and musicians. People who had used it included the writer Rod Temperton who formed the band Heatwave but became world renowned as the writer of tracks on Michael Jackson's biggest hit album 'Thriller'. You may recall his *'Blame it on the Boogie'*.

I was told by his mate Alan Kirk who was keyboards player in Jimmy James & The Vagabonds and has his own studio at Dronfield, near Sheffield, that Michael Jackson's producer Quincy Jones had already chosen Rod's songs for inclusion on Thriller but they'd slipped up by not signing him up to a publishing contract before they'd gone to the expense of recording his songs for the album.

This meant Rod was in an amazing negotiating position to make himself rich. Indeed, he became very, very, stinking rich thank to Thriller and he had his own great band too Heatwave.

Others who made their way in the music business by using Fairview for their demos were Sheffield rockers Def Leppard.

My Rainmaker demo must have had a good vibe because another record company at the time called Anchor Records also wanted to sign me on the strength of it. "We've played it to our staff, and they love it," said the chief A&R guy. A&R for the uninitiated that is the artistes and repertoire department.

But it was CBS I chose to record that first 'Rainmaker' single. They put me in a studio with musicians, but not on this first recording venture with the orchestra that I've mentioned earlier, but with part of an established band called *Argent* and these were lovely guys, who'd had a big hit with a track called *'Hold Your Head Up'*. However, they were rock musicians and when I heard them play my pop song, I instinctively knew it just wasn't going to work. The vibe wasn't there. In the end to try and give the song some tempo and to lose a drag we felt the song had, it was speeded up at the final mix.

Unfortunately, this speeding-up made my already high-pitched rendition unbelievably higher so much so that famous pop critic of her time Caroline Coon in Sounds who reviewed the song said it sounded as if a great white shark had got me by the privates – *Jaws* the film was on release at the time.

I thought the record 'B' side was a better representation of what I could do. That B side was *'Mind Blowing Love'* and became record of the week on quite a few UK radio stations. Unsurprisingly to me Rainmaker bombed, apart from in Portugal where it was listened to a lot and sold well. It was suggested to me that this was so because Portugal at that time was in dire need of rain and suffering a drought. I imagined the population dancing to it hoping it would bring rain falling upon parched land.

My song title, if not the song itself, found prominence though not long after on that same CBS label I was signed to when The Wombles released a song called 'Rainmaker'. Not the same song, just a coincidence, eh? As a gimmick for my own Rainmaker, I should too have been a woolly creature that cleared litter off Wimbledon Common for the launch.

At my signing of the contract at CBS I was informed that I would be called Alan Childe – they smartly gave me a new name – and they had the idea that I would succeed the heart-throb teen idol of the time David Essex. I was pencil thin with long, long hair and best described as androgynous which is what every successful pop star e.g. Bowie and Bolan looked like.

I had married straight out of school and being a good catholic was three children up before birth control entered my thoughts. While with CBS it wasn't possible to pursue music full time as I had a family to support.

The record label never knew I had a wife and children and I didn't tell them because they didn't ask but they probably thought I didn't look capable of it either. In those days they did rather like pop stars to be accessible to their fans – and that meant being single and available.

Anyway, at a meeting at CBS with the accounts chief, who bizarrely was wearing something like the attire you'd wear crossing a desert, I wasn't represented by a lawyer. Their legal eagle ate me alive. They offered me 13% on my record sales which with stars in my eyes I readily accepted. It was going to be the shortest meeting on record.

I knew 13 per cent was amazing and accepted immediately their generosity towards a poor Northern boy. What I didn't know was that I was supposed to barter with them and then they would have offered me an advance on which I might be able to live and in return I would bring my 13% rate down to a more realistic rate of say 6%.

I had signed something like a five-album deal. If all my albums reached number one at 13% I could have been owning CBS Records further down the line. As it was circumstances decreed that I never did make one album with them. Along came The Clash and they no longer had to pay for orchestras to provide backing for songs composed in bedrooms by poor Northern boys.

There were times in London when opportunities arose to live a little like a pop star – but with my good catholic upbringing I resisted.

I recall once going down the stairway of the CBS Soho Square office and passing this interesting looking, attractive young lady who was accompanied by what looked like a security team. I threw a Jaffa orange her way and she caught it and threw it back. Such fun was this that a full-scale fruit slinging match might have occurred. We laughed said hi to each other. I swear sparks flew. By the time I'd got to the foot of the stairs, one of her team from the top of the stairs had chased down after me to say: "Roseanne would like it if you'd join her at a nightclub tonight?"

I was due to head home in my brother's old jalopy parked outside the studio. With just a little regret I said thanks but no thanks.

There are crossroads in life and if I had accepted Roseanne's offer and if we had hit it off at that nightclub quite as spectacularly as we had done over one simple Jaffa orange then Johnny Cash might one day have been my father-in-law, because the girl in question was his daughter Roseanne, now of course a big country star in the US.

Rumour travels fast in show business. When I next visited CBS A & R department the first thing they asked was: "How's it going with Roseanne?" They weren't joking.

It would have been a publicity coop for CBS if a poor unknown pop singer from the North of England had been dating Johnny Cash's daughter – Johnny Cash incidentally having sold 90,000 million records worldwide.

There would have been plenty of photo opportunities for Roseanne and I.

I would have taken her down a coal mine and shown her around a steelworks giving her a better idea of my roots and where I might have ended up working if I hadn't signed to CBS.

All I knew about Roseanne's dad at the time was that he encouraged an outlaw image and you wouldn't want to get on the wrong side of him.

I saw the look of disappointment on the faces of the A&R guys when I said I wasn't dating Roseanne. The colour drained from their faces. If only… they were thinking.

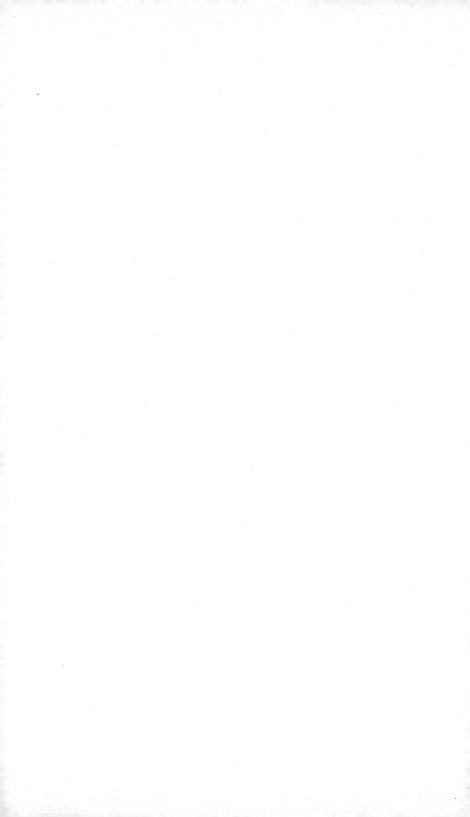

CHAPTER SIXTEEN

FACING UP TO TRAGEDY

I interpose in my writing to tell you that I read just the other day in a newspaper a plea from a mental health expert that those who help deal with tragic occurrences should be given post traumatic psychological help. I'm overdue for a lot of help then.

As a newspaper reporter you deal with tragedy all the time – it never stops coming.

There is seldom a no news day or dull moment in journalism. I used to turn stories around quickly.

While working as chief reporter in the New Forest for the Bournemouth Echo I was heavily engaged in reporting the aftermath of the Christchurch British Legion coach crash which killed 19. I went to Bristol to cover the trial of the coach driver. I attended the inquests of the victims and even attended funerals. It was touching, moving and I got to know the survivors and feel their loss at losing their friends and relatives.

I was already battle hardened to do what I did then because while working on The Sheffield Journal as its editor, and doing almost every other duty too, including tea boy, I covered the aftermath of the Hillsborough disaster.

I was there on the day the current Prime Minister Margaret Thatcher walked the death terraces of Leppings Lane to see for herself the crumpled crash barriers, bent by the pressure of the heaving crowd that day.

Ninety-seven died on the day of the Hillsborough tragedy and there were 766 injuries. I watched like millions of others did as it unfolded on TV on a Saturday afternoon. I lived just a few miles from the stadium itself.

I went into work the following day to get organised and by Monday morning I was on the job interviewing survivors and reporting stories from those trapped in the dark tunnel at Hillsborough who survived being trampled to death as panicking fans attempted to escape the crush. I interviewed kind and willing householders on the streets outside the football ground who had gone to the aid of distressed football fans streaming from the ground.

People were still in tears and mourning. It was like a black cloud had parked itself over Sheffield and wouldn't move away. Blame for what happened was being bandied about.

For many forthcoming weeks following the disaster our newspapers stories were Hillsborough, Hillsborough, Hillsborough. I can't say that it didn't have a big effect on me as it soaked in.

The thing about reporting is that you get the job done and you try not to get involved so that you do the job properly. You detach and see things from the other side of the lens. Here's the moral dilemma of the press photographer. Does he try and save people in a train crash or does he keeping shooting his camera, doing his job so the world will know about the tragedy?

That's a tough one.

He will have been schooled that he should keep taking pictures. Maybe the best journalists are the ones who can detach from emotions at times like these and just write what they see without involving themselves in the action. I knew all about detaching from emotions as a child I did it and now I was doing it as an adult as a reporter. I was a sightseer. I was there on the periphery of happening things asking why they had occurred to tell others. You are trusted to do that job. You must be brave enough to tell it as it is, though some people will threaten you with personal extinction for some facts you have hold of if you publish them.

In the profession one of the toughest jobs in journalism is 'the door knock'.

I did it many, many times when I worked on early morning calls on various newspapers. On early morning police calls you pick up the accidents, for instance the young lad who had been mowed down on his way to school by a lorry driver near his house and killed.

In the early hours of the morning, you scrape the frost from your windscreen and head to the boy's house. Then you summon the courage to door knock. The parents come to the door in tears. You wonder why you do this job.

"I'm very sorry to hear what has happened to your son, I'm from the Echo I wonder if you could spare me just 10 minutes so that I can talk to you about son?"

At this point many a journalist will get the door slammed in his face and that's that. You walk away. You don't harass the bereaved. They have enough grief to cope with without you pressurising and upsetting them further.

I was lucky, if you'd call it that. I never did have the door slammed in my face. I was always respectful, and I was either invited inside to talk or if not I would conduct my interview from the doorstep.

I always told parents that what I wrote would be a tribute in the newspaper to their son or daughter. I also told them it was better, much safer if they gave me their account because then we could be sure it was accurate. If we went to neighbours on the street or the kid's friends for our story, who knows what they'd tell us? We didn't want to publish hearsay stuff from people who might claim to have known the child but didn't.

On one of my first jobs on calls at the *Sheffield Star* I was assigned by the news desk to cover a bad stabbing at one of the city's high-rise flats. We had no firm address and I when I got there the high rise loomed upwards until I lost sight of it as it faded into a grey very foggy early morning sky. It looked about as tall as a Manhattan skyscraper.

I didn't go up in the lift, I was always scared of getting trapped. My fears though were well founded. Lifts on this estate were always breaking down and users were trapped inside them, sometimes for hours. To me it would have been akin to being buried alive. I did fire calls in the mornings, and the fire service told me they visited the lifts often to rescue trapped residents when lifts broke down.

With no clues to the knifing, I must have legged it to the fifth floor. It paid to be fit. I began knocking on doors. There was no-one around at this time of morning to answer my questions. It was a needle in a haystack job.

I rang the news desk to tell them my task looked hopeless. No mobile phones in those days so I had to return to ground level to use the one telephone box. That box seemed to have most of the world's graffiti scrawled upon it and stank of pee. I was a miracle the phone was still useable; they often weren't because of mindless vandalism.

Typically, I was told to stay in pursuit of the story by the desk. Was I really supposed to door knock 600 homes?

I went back up and was on the fifth or sixth floor knocking on doors. Nothing.

By this time, I was looking down, not up. I had noticed I had a shoelace undone. I bent down to tie it and spotted on the ground... blood.

That morning I followed a trail of blood right to the door of where the knife attack took place, and I got my story.

Incidentally, White News Agency in Sheffield got itself into big trouble by reporting the Hillsborough football tragedy during which 97 fans died. The story they distributed was the controversial one that Liverpool football fans had behaved intolerably and had been drunk and caused the disaster. It proved to be untrue.

I knew reporters working on that agency. Good lads. Newspaper reporters always sailed close to the wind with what they wrote and but if you managed to balance a story by getting both sides of an argument you were okay. Allow the reader after getting both sides of an argument to decide who was the bad guy and who the good.

That story though condemned the Liverpool fans who weren't given a voice to defend themselves.

CHAPTER SEVENTEEN

GENDER FLUIDITY AND THE REST

Isn't it great that children growing up today will be able to openly tell the world who they are without facing prejudice or reprisal.

Hopefully future generations of children will be able to grow up and express to others who they are and feel comfortable with how they feel, think and how they identify themselves to others.

In an ideal world they will know how best they function and fit in with others and hopefully how to live their lives to the full instead of being told, as was in the past in relatively recent history as far as gender is concerned, that there are only two categories by which they can define themselves, either male or female.

I'll take two of those relatively new labels doing the rounds and ascribe them to myself in the way I think and feel, and they are gender fluid and non-binary.

You who are reading this might be a cupiosexual, grey romantic, androsexual or one of 57 other categories that better define who you are and help you feel comfortable in your own skin. You might be straight down the middle heterosexual, or thought you were but you were never quite sure? Now you can check out the labels and see if there's a match more suited to how

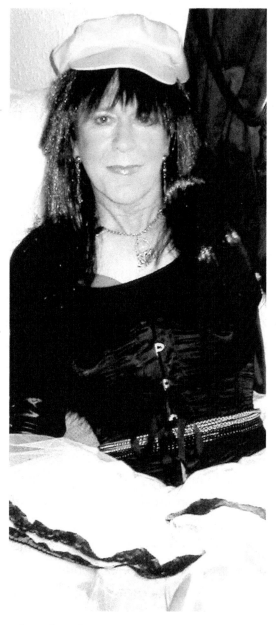

Alan chart hit in Greece as Angel Deelite

you feel or think. You might re-align yourself and find greater happiness in knowing and accepting who you are rather than being conveniently boxed by others.

As always, times are changing.

I smiled when I saw a story headlined in a national newspaper today in 2022 '*Less Than Half of Cambridge Students Are Heterosexual*'. A similar survey at Oxford University produced a similar result.

If you think that self-identification or the right to choose to be who you feel and think you are, is going away or that labels are bunkum, you're just not moving with the times.

It's confusing and challenging to some to accept the differences of others.

Many older people are set in their ways and cannot grasp new thinking, but thankfully not all.

Opponents of new freedoms of expression offering inclusivity for all can struggle to understand why things must change, while others just refuse to listen or are unwilling to accommodate. That is usually their loss in the long run.

Some don't want to share the freedoms and advantages they have with those they consider lesser or unworthy individuals. Some are indoctrinated by dubious religious teaching to think the way they do. Progress demands from everyone the opening of hearts, sharing, compassion and a willingness to change and embrace differences.

New terminologies for the new age hopefully mean no-one is left out anymore or repressed because of how they feel or think.

It will allow them to distinguish and meet others like themselves, to not be isolated and to learn more about themselves.

When the majority rules and minorities of all kinds based on say gender or colour of skin are looked upon unfavourably by the rulers you get oppression, you get Russia and China. You get the opposite of freedom. You get your mind made up for you.

History shows enlightenment leads to celebration. Humans, providing their intention is to do no harm, can live and thrive together and celebrate their differences. They can also fight injustice together. They can be inclusive and fair. Minorities coming together can make up a new and hopefully fairer majority.

Two of my great personal successes were achieved when I allowed what I'll describe as my feminine side to take charge. Never accuse me of not being versatile. For one project I wore a dress a wig and make-up and sang and performed as *Angel Deelite* – and on another occasion I was on stage as Karen Carpenter, my favourite all time female vocalist, one half of the fabulous Carpenters.

First, I'll tell you about *Angel Deelite*.

This appeared on my JohnnyDysfunctional.com website telling the unlikeliest of stories.

JOHNNY reached No2 in the Greece charts with his co-written song 'Big Romance' and it involved him in a sex-swap.

He glammed-up to become Angel Deelite and unbelievably but true was only kept from the top of the charts by US megastar Shakira.

Here is the chart...

Θέση	Προηγ. Θέση	Τραγούδι - Καλλιτέχνης	
1	1	**La tortura** - *Shakira*	●
2	4	**Big romance** - *Angel Deelite*	▲
3	2	**You're beautiful** - *James Blunt*	▼
4	7	**Till there was you** - *Rachel Star*	▲
5	3	**Diamonds from Sierra Leone** - *Kanye West & Jay Z*	▼
6	5	**Feel good Inc** - *Gorillaz*	▼
7	6	**Mamakossa** - *Back To Basics vs Ktf*	▼
8	8	**Coracao** - *Jerry Ropero & Denis The Menace*	●
9	10	**Hate it or love it** - *The Game feat. 50 Cent*	▲
10	9	**Don't phunk with my heart** - *Black Eyed Peas*	▼

Chart position

Mind you, Johnny had no complaints because Angel Deelite (sitting at No2 in the chart) was way ahead in Greece of Coldplay, Oasis, Black Eyed Peas and Kanye West and Jay Z.

Johnny said: "I suppose Shakira deserved the number one spot because she was authentically sensational... but I reckon I ran her pretty close thanks to my make-up lady and dresser. We nearly got the number one slot," he said.

Johnny added: "When the label released the song everybody thought it was a female singer so I did a quick switch to give the public what it expected," he said.

FACING SURGERY? DON'T BE A SCAREDY CAT

As I mentioned, I usually go under the name of Johnny Dysfunctional to write and record and not Alan Childe as CBS has named me, nor Alan Charnley nor Marmaduke Jinks my novel writing pen name. This was another of my pop creations – *Angel Deelite*.

If this cancer takes me in the end... as it might. I'm laying claim to having one of the most gender fluid voices around and there will be recordings to prove it if anyone chooses to listen to them!

Try *'Love's Arrived'* in my best falsetto under the name of Sydney Brook on Soundcloud.

https://soundcloud.com/johnnydysfunctional/loves-arrived-sydney-brook

Since quite early childhood I realized in myself signs that I was an internal mix of heart and mind of the masculine and feminine. I never did have the words to know or describe what was going on inside of me or who or what I was, but I've always been grateful for the gift it has given me.

It has given me an insight into the male and female psyche and enabled me to have conversations and a closeness with others I might never have achieved without it.

So why haven't I flaunted it and let it be, so to speak?

Well, I have, in plain sight, on stage.

I might have been a scaredy cat without using that front, without wearing the mask of performance or maybe I just never wanted fuss and enjoy my privacy as most of us do. But of course, for many there is another reason they hold back. Some are children of their time and in my own time had I owned up to being non-binary I would have been shunned, called a pervert or been at the back end of the queue for opportunities and no doubt I'd have had to deal with the isolation it brought too. It's unbelievable but true. I'd had quite enough of isolation.

I think its great new terminology exists to describe those in the past who have struggled to fit into this world because of their differences. It is good to be able to speak of how we feel and think, it is good for all to be able to do so. People have been too often condemned to live their lives as a lie, denying their true selves out of fear and fear alone.

Don't be a scaredy cat.

Talking to people in general of either gender I know I baffle them sometimes with what I know about the opposite gender.

I'll give you an example I was once speaking to a man about his girlfriend problem and though we'd only just met he unloaded on me. This is not uncommon. Men and women do randomly. I can go deeply into things with men on topics they usually don't talk about or are reluctant to do so. The man I am referring to in this instance said I don't know why I'm telling you all of this. It was because I knew the right questions to ask, and I had constructive answers. I see things from and speak from a man's perspective as well as a woman's.

A woman in the bar overhearing that conversation approached me afterwards and introduced herself as a therapist. She said 'wow' I wish my husband could talk to me like you just talked to him. My gender fluidity has given me insight.

I once read that Indian tribes in America had a special tepee for someone of my ilk. In some tribes the gender fluid was considered the wise ones and seeing 'both sides' gave advice to both men and women. They were treated with great respect.

I don't have a tepee, but I was a Samaritan for five years giving advice. I was very comfortable helping both troubled men and women.

While writing with the cancer charities I often interviewed women recovering or fighting from breast cancer. One-woman colleague who sat next to me commented one day: "I don't know how you can ask those questions to women about their breasts."

"What do you mean. I'm asking them about how they deal with their breast cancer?" I told her.

"You do it so well, but you are a man. I don't understand."

I was being a compassionate human being. I understand it better myself now. I am, as I say, non-binary. I was not embarrassed because I was listening and understanding their feelings and predicaments. I was empathizing.

Hiding in plain sight? Here's more of the story of Angel Deelite.

While working in Christchurch, near Bournemouth, as a reporter, covering speedway and winning Southern Sports Writer of the Year with one of the judges being the late David English, Editor of *The Daily Mail*, my musical journey took another turn when I met up with Kevin Charge who played keyboards and been a musical director for some top American outfits who came over to play their music in the UK.

Kevin, a joy to work with and a natural fit musically to me, had also had the privilege and claim to fame of once playing along with Stevie Wonder on a piano in a pub after his gig concluded.

I don't know if Kevin was the one sat at the bass side of the piano or sat at the tinkly end. Forgot to ask him that one.

With Kevin I recorded a song – in a high register and many thought it was a female singing our song *Big Romance*. Anyway, this song, as can be seen from the chart above went all the way to No2 kept off the top spot only by a sexy female singer by the name of Shakira.

However, our song was well ahead in the charts of big names like of Coldplay Jay Z, Kanye West, Oasis Black Eyed Peas and the like.

We posted a story that it was a female singer on the song, a girl busker we had 'discovered' singing on Bournemouth Pier and how we had since lost touch with her. We sent out an SOS to the world in order that Alan and Kevin could be reunited with the girl we had called *Angel Deelite*. All baloney of course and done because Alan and Angel could never be on stage together, for an obvious reason.

After an amazing long summer chart positioning our song was then stolen and during the winter pirated by an Easter European company. Our publishing company had lost track of its where-abouts. It also ended up on an album that was sold in France. We were on that album with artistes like Elton John. Kevin and I didn't see a penny from its sales of which there must have been plenty, but neither must Elton have seen a single pound for his efforts.

Now my other successful appearance on stage as a female as I mentioned was as Karen Carpenter. I'm sure there were some in those few-hundreds of people who saw the shows who weren't entirely sure whether it wasn't a female singing up on that stage. I was told that was the case by some of my friends seated in the audience.

Karen's brother Richard, the other half of *The Carpenters* duo said famously Karen was impossible to copy vocally because she was a one off. Agreed but I got as close as I could get.

The shows went exceedingly well judging by the audience reaction.

Yes, stage gave me an outlet and with hindsight it did take a lot of courage to go out and play Karen in that self-penned musical called '*Come Back to Blackpool, Karen Carpenter*'.

Before I wrote the script, I never believed that the great Karen Carpenter, she with the velvet voice, had sung in Blackpool, she was more likely to have sung on the moon in my estimation than Blackpool, but I was to discover much later that uncannily she had.

The plot I wrote for the show was about an Elvis Presley tribute impersonator, played by me, who one night hears the haunting voice of Karen coming from a juke box. From then on this stage character Stephen Oliphant, yes, played by me, feels it's his destiny to promote Karen's music and her voice with a tribute act.

I got to sing all of Karen's big hits.

Karen died tragically from anorexia and is my favourite female vocalist by a long stretch.

Hers was a character I could lose myself in and the shows were such a great pleasure in which to act and to sing. It was a two hander with Deirdre Costello an actor who had a long career in films like *The Full Monty* and TV and radio roles. She played Oliphant's brassy wife.

Deirdre was so enamoured by the show she believed it wouldn't be long before we were invited to switch on the Blackpool illuminations. I sang all Karen's hits and to dress as The Carpenter's star did was simplicity itself. I wore a long dark wig and long hippy dress. Karen was 'sold' to the public by her management as 'the innocent girl next door'. Those dresses had shoulder pads and the long dark hair formed curtains around her pale face.

I sung all her hits and it transferred from a pub venue to Buxton's Pavilion theatre with its full lighting and effect.

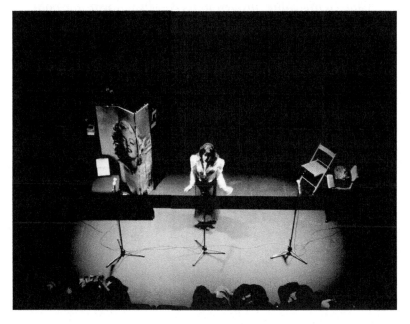

As Karen Carpenter

The review said

The Grove Hotel

This is a new writing by the very talented Johnny Dysfunctional and Deirdre Costello. Whilst not purporting to be an impersonation of Karen Carpenter, Johnny's portrayal was spookily close – well done and keeping the singing voice going throughout. It was great hearing the great songs again and being reminded of Karen's tragically short life.

We are taken through the rough patch that Johnny and Chazza are going through to its conclusion which is both funny and sad and very well played.

The audience was singing along and really appreciative of the trip down memory lane. We even had a cameo appearance from a Beatle and Elvis!

Thank you this was a good fun show with great songs well performed.

Linda McAlinden

From there the Karen show was performed in Oxford and in Bournemouth.

I think I did Karen proud. I must confess and I'd like to do it again sometime.

Anyway, I sing and write with either my male or female head switched on. With me that's just the way it is. Even in the dim, dark distant past I used to do what is now considered to be fair

172

in the cause of inclusivity I was consciously avoided pronouns in my song writing that would indicate to others I was a man singing about a woman or vice versa.

It was love between two people I wrote about. I wanted my song to touch the hearts of people listening whoever they were. In that respect I was ahead of my time. I wrote in the way I did because I felt it was right.

I've used my late dad's name Sydney, a name used by both genders to record female original songs as *Sydney Brook*. I have recorded and released an album '*Unique*' and a London producer put out as a single from it called '*World Peace*'. I haven't yet promoted the Sydney album. I should.

https://open.spotify.com/track/0xvygXcmKwGswhq68Kfutk

This is an expression, a part of myself and I've decided to tell you about here because my diagnosis of cancer means I might not be around anyway when this book comes out though I hope I am.

I came from an era whereby if you were different there were blokes with overloads of testosterone with bike chains for brains who would gang up on you in an instant to either ridicule, beat you up or abuse you. Other kids joined in because they wanted to be on the winning side, and the bullies reigned and got away with it for so long. It is incredible that the law of the land supported that kind of thinking, intolerance, and hate. It still goes on, of course and especially in other countries and always will.

To live in peace and have the freedom to be who you are on the understanding you respect others too is what most people would agree upon to live happily ever after in this complex world.

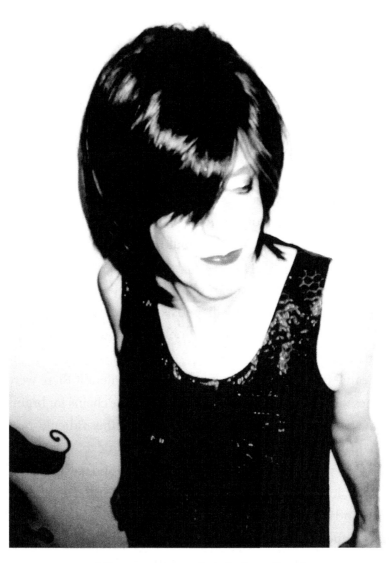

Alan as pop creation Sydney Brook

It is a complex world that does hold simple answers if we seek them out and show compassion.

I love the musical journey and I have never been materialistic. I have always felt that my songs through melody and words expressed strong sentiments. Some who have heard these songs appreciate the emotional content and take something from them and tell me so. Job done. Then there are others who will listen with blank faces, those emotionally tuned out, those with an absence of emotional intelligence who miss a song's whole point. That's life. I write songs of love, loss and more. Music can be magic.

I hope that if my late dad Syd looks down from a celestial palace where maybe he plays splendidly a harp, that he enjoys the songs I write too.

CHAPTER EIGHTEEN

MOTHER & CHILD REUNION ON FACEBOOK AFTER 50 YEARS

I wrote my story about a mother and child reunion after an estrangement of more than 50 years, a reunion that took place on the social network site Facebook of all places. I thought the story in the following form suitable for a magazine before I decided instead to go the whole hog and write a bit of a book.

The magazine story read like this.

THE GHOST OF MY DAD

My mother's love I never understood as a child or an adult – and I only learned about the truths of my own confusion when she was aged 91 and I was in my late 60's and we broke a 50-years plus estrangement to share between us tens of thousands of words messaging over Facebook.

With fingers affected by arthritis she had mastered an I-pad and got in touch.

Following around 18 month of messaging we met just the once to make our peace before her death aged 93.

The relationship with my mother as I was growing up was as intense at times as it was distant and so very confusing. It was only very late in my life after our Facebook reunion that I was able to connect the dots and understand why it was how it was and to finally come to terms with what happened to cause our rift.

The circumstances that prevented my mother and I having a normal relationship were out of the ordinary, to say the least.

It began when the Americans dropped their second atomic bomb on the Japanese fishing port of Nagasaki in 1945.

It heralded the end of the Second World War and that was when my father-to-be was dispatched from the UK with the Royal Engineers to help rebuild the flattened remains of that Japanese city where tens of thousands of men woman and children were killed.

When my father Syd returned from Japan his romance with Judith continued and soon my mother fell pregnant with me.

But Sid had brought back from Japan a legacy of War – a cancer caused by the nuclear radiation. Soon it riddled his body, and my mother was to tell me how doctors experimented on him with the permission of his father, knowing that he would die anyway.

My mother said the hospital ward in the West Midlands she visited to see Syd was full of returned soldiers from Japan dying from the same cancer.

After Syd's death my mother was alone and thrown into poverty and she told me that one night she decided to kill us both by gassing us to death using the oven.

She took a walk with me and came to her senses just in time she told me when she looked down upon her baby – me – in a pram.

She re-married soon after to Terry who became my stepdad and I recall he and I enjoyed playing games when I was younger, but once that stopped there was, little in common between us. I became a solitary child and immersed myself in my imagination. I wrote stories and songs from an early age.

During my childhood, my mother at times would burst into my bedroom room and hold me tightly. She would also shout warnings to Terry to 'keep his hands off me'. At other times she would enter my room and angrily accuse me of 'coming between her and Terry'. She said she would deal with me for being naughty so that he wouldn't. There were times she was slap happy with me.

I knew nothing of why she behaved so erratically towards me until I was about 10. Then she told me Terry was not my real father. She came into my bedroom to tell me just that – and then left without explaining further. I recall replying: "But he is my dad."

Who my real father was, was not spoken about any further by either my mother or my stepdad. Syd didn't exist – but he did, as a ghost.

It turned out that my mother had been deeply in love with Syd and married Terry on the rebound because he could look after her. Terry was jealous of her relationship with Syd even though he was dead and the child that I was, was Terry and Judy's constant reminder of Syd. Terry burned all the photos of Syd, but how much resentment at times he felt towards me, Syd's living reminder whenever they argued it is difficult to judge.

Bottom line is that my late father was a ghost in the houses where we lived.

My mother kept a tight rein on her emotions about the loss of Syd and the abuse she had suffered as a young girl, that I knew nothing about. I grew unable to speak of my emotions and confused about the father I never knew. I had lived in an emotional lockdown.

Weeks before her death and aged 93 she told me that Syd had come to her in a dream. She was still in love with him.

That was comforting for me to know. I hadn't wanted my dad forgotten though I had never met him.

Many readers will know how difficult it is not to know anything about a birth father or mother. My difficulty extended to not knowing why my mother and I could not share a bond. I think I learned to keep my emotions buried and for a very long time my only release for these emotions was through my songs and my stories.

I like to think my mum and Syd are now reunited and now I have grown-up and understand more I have no

problem about Terry joining the pair of them to laugh
about it all!

Of all the reunions achieved through Facebook, the one that involved my mother and I, she 91 and terminally dying from cancer, must stand-out as the most unusual of them all.

There she was technologically adept and in touch not only with me on the social network using an I Pad but now telling me regularly in messages that she was 'ready to go'. To die, she meant.

"Why am I still here when everyone around me has died?" she would write.

Another message read:

> *"I'm not grumbling I do have mobility scooter to get to the*
> *shops. I do have terminal cancer which I'm on drugs for*
> *but I'm not grumbling because my life is almost over now*
> *and I'm ready for what comes next."*
>
> *At ninety-one I've had some bad times! And fought back*
> *and some good times learned a lot About life. Buried a*
> *lot of family and friends and sometimes wonder why I'm*
> *still here.*

I must admit that had I not by then trained and worked as a Samaritan listening to all kinds of problems from all kinds of people, I might not have coped so well with the torrent of upset and information coming my way. At times communicating with her was like walking over eggshells.

181

There were times had I not been disciplined when I might have rushed to judgement about her disclosures resulting in battle lines being drawn and the healing process being halted. Do not be judgmental with callers was the first rule of The Samaritans and I followed that advice.

Now I was tip toeing my way to discovering as much as I could about Syd, my mum's past and myself and hopefully without upsetting too greatly a 91-year-old very poorly woman who though she was desperately ill was as bright as a button mentally.

I was most surprised that we did eventually broker our peace because in the past and before this Facebook contact, I feared that speaking with my mother would prove pointless. I anticipated at such great age she may have lost her faculties as so many older people tragically do.

My mother's letters written to me in the past were at the core of my believing I was not loved or understood by her. It seemed most of the time when I was growing up, she didn't want to know who I was.

I came to believe I was a token of my late father's love and I had been integrated into her new family and that had been achieved by her striking a deal with her new husband. Her sacrifice to him was to block out any conversation or references to my true father as the pair forged their future. Their deal and intention had been to move on without ever again acknowledging the reality of my mother's past life and there would be no more talk of her former love. That deal would have been a further bolt on the door wherein were kept the secrets my mother already stored. Who knows what she did or didn't tell Terry. Years and years later my mother had nursed Terry when he suffered vascular dementia, until his death.

I remember a pal when I was in my 30's expressing this next viewpoint and for some reason his words stayed with me because they were so heartfelt. Now that late time of life my pal was referring to has arrived at my door: "Old age is such a cruel and horrible thing. I never want to be old," he had said shaking his head morbidly. Take credit Francis Batt long standing reporter on *The Windsor& Eton Express* and TV film buff. I hope wherever you are you found the elixir to youth.

It's true that until we reach what we consider to be an old age to us, we never know the full horror of the number of illnesses and cancers that lie in waiting for most if not all of us.

Any vestiges of that immortal feeling of eternal youth have long vanished by this autumnal stage of life and we expect our remaining winters to be harsh. A newly adopted philosophy of devil-may-care about what may happen next or of resignation to fate is now called for and necessary. You are nothing now more than one of the many enlisted soldiers of your generation about to be called to the frontline – maybe you'll even end up on life support!

If one disease or illness doesn't remove you from life, then another surely will. You may conjecture on which malady you'd accept in preference to another. I used to reflect on that even when I was a kid. 'Would I rather go deaf than blind?' I considered. Oh well, it may be both now, you meekly and bleakly accept. Pass the wine bottle.

Probably the worst thing is to sink into depression.

Stay positive! Don't be a scaredy cat.

My mother died having already been told she had terminal breast cancer. Can it be ruled out that the sun lamp treatment I mentioned in an earlier chapter all those years ago did not contribute to her death? No, it can't, but conveniently it can't be proved that it did either.

Despite our long correspondence on Facebook, for a year going on two, mother and I only met each other in the flesh just the once before she died. I spontaneously decided I should just drop in on her without invitation at her sheltered housing flat.

Call it intuition that told me it was finally the time to bite the bullet and to travel and see her. I figured she couldn't have had long left, and she had kept pushing that point home in her messaging. I went along to see her with my wife Gillian. It had an amusing start as I was to meet the vitriolic tongue of my mother.

She hadn't been in her flat when we arrived, but a passer-by on the corridor outside saw us as we knocked on her door.

"She's with the hairdresser having her hair done. It's the room down the corridor," she directed.

I went to that room instead after knocking on the door. She had her back to me. I saw her face in the mirror staring back at mine. She turned in her chair and the hairdresser paused styling my mum's white hair before my mother stood up and after pulling a towel away. She looked at me fiercely.

I said nothing but smiled at her.

"What are you doing in here. Who are you? Get out. Get out," she ordered me squeakily and feistily. I recognised that voice. That take no prisoners style of hers.

I still said nothing.

Then it dawned upon her.

"Alan. Is that my son Alan?" she quizzed and then we both walked towards each other and hugged. Fifty years bridged in one moment. Then the hostess in her took over. We were escorted back to her flat where she made us both a hot drink. She was introduced to Gillian.

Mother was soon reminiscing rather a lot, especially on her favourite topic, the time when she was having the time of life, in the army and 'free' she said. That time also included meeting the love of her life, my dad Syd, though he was not spoken of at this meeting – she had in previous correspondence said that Syd was 'slow' – probably shy – in that she had waited so long for him to ask her out. Women didn't go on the front foot and ask a man out if she fancied him back in those days.

In the lead-up to that day's meet up, over those two inter-vening years of corresponding we had debated, fixed things and fallen out on Facebook so nothing on this day would be too taboo to discuss now – one of us could not, would not ambush the other. Mother asked Gillian about her health, which had not been good over a long period.

On hearing how poorly she had been and how often Gillian was bedridden, she turned to me and said: "You must be like a dog on heat!"

That was a typically 'sensitive' remark from my mother. I recall after my first marriage to Anne, when I was in my 20's. I had remarked: "I wish we'd employed a professional photographer to cover my wedding."

She turned to me and replied in all seriousness: "But why? Neither of you are oil paintings."

She wasn't one for boosting my self-esteem, however the fact that my looks didn't apparently appeal to her didn't prevent me in my mid 20's from signing a major recording company contract with CBS Records, the American communication giant.

I should have reminded her that they viewed me as a potential androgynous heart throb and wanted to market me as such. I was to be groomed as a successor to its UK pop star of that day David Essex, who they complained to me was giving them trouble. Of course, I'd never had that conversation with her.

Incidentally, as far as I could gather David Essex only wanted more control over his career and to record more of his own material. Any pop stars in that era were micro-managed and it's likely they still are today. I was more suited to what came next which was the devil may care punk movement, but when The Clash did come along at that label, CBS didn't anymore have to spend great amounts on studio session musicians and orchestral arrangements, and I was unceremoniously dropped. If you are a fan of The Clash thank me. I made way for them.

What was amusing was when The Clash parked their vehicle next to our old jalopy outside the recording studios at Whitfield Street, London, they had a registration plate on a car belonging to one of them that depicted their band name. We poor Northerners couldn't afford a personalised registration plate.

But from The Clash back to my mother. We were together in a room for the first time in 50 years or so.

I never knew how or what my mother saw in me or if she ever noted my exploits as a marathon runner, a performer singer songwriter or as a journalist, as thin as these exploits might appear to some.

I had at an early stage of my life introduced her to my songs asking for her feedback. Her response was always 'that's nice'.

'That's nice' she said to every single one of my new songs. And after every listening, I recall she used to leave the room quickly. In the end, always with the same thing occurring, I felt it wasn't worth bothering. She had a record collection which included Mario Lanza and Petula Clark so her choice of recordings might have once been an influence on my writing. They might have been because I'd played them often enough over and over again, limited by choice and no money to buy others. It was me wearing those discs out the most, alone in my room. Subsequently any one of my own original songs I played her had she really listened might have had carried perhaps a hint of a similar pretty melody she already liked that could have sent her into raptures had she switched off the vacuum cleaner to listen to a song at least twice! The vac cleaner though won the day.

Another possibility was that mum had shut down on listening to love songs and after all, what did I know writing love songs at my tender age, she might have been thinking. The lyrical content would have amounted to nothing compared to her own tragic experience!

It was rare during those early years she broke off housework. She was like a hamster on a wheel. You may think I should have been grateful for the 'nice' feedback on each song? She could easily have said something vindictive and destroyed me there and then with one of her off-the-cuff remarks as sometimes seemed to be her want.

When I recall the ire of her letters sent to me before we became estranged, 'you will die in the gutter' and 'you're no son of mine' being the worst, I have since wondered if mother existed somewhere on the autistic scale.

Our Facebook link up is best described as a massive correspondence between the two of us. It went from exchanging niceties to occasional bouts of upsetting home truths delivered from both sides.

It was the coming together of something that had never been forged tightly in the first place. It was a rocky communion. Ours had been a mother and son arrangement in name only. The band aids that sustained whatever passed as a relationship in our early years when I was passive to her whims and temper without question were ripped off. The scales fell from our eyes.

The result of this was that our Facebook contact broke off from time to time with either one of us anguishing on what had been said. These 'splits' could last for a few weeks while we both ruminated on what we had written and its effect on one or the other of us. We were both grown up and were tough enough though to return to the fray and finish what we had started.

As might be imagined, we both had differing accounts or memories of our past and how we had felt and why we did what we did or didn't do many years ago when I was a child and she the parent. Those times leave deep scars. We both had heavy bolted doors that needed to creak open. And we did it. When a

Facebook impasse, an awkward or hurtful interruption occurred and a 'breather' was taken there would follow from my mother a token letter of peace by post in which she self-chastised, telling me how she had always felt she wasn't good enough, that she'd been ill educated, but always these letters revealed more information.

She swung from knowing it all and being the font of all wisdom to the role of a martyr expressing herself in the lowest of low self-esteem. But was her response seeking pity or was she just using her regular route out of jams and what she really thought was that I was the cause of all problems in her life?

Deep down I began to see how insecure she was behind the bombastic outer shell. In one of these letter's, she described herself as a pig. At her funeral service she was called 'charismatic'. Maybe chameleon was a better description.

However, on Facebook she was giving me more and more information about my past that I had previously been denied knowledge of.

"If you want I could explain about Syd but must be your choice it was very hard at the time! I did love him deeply and it affected me deeply but time heals x"

I responded: *"Ah, that is lovely to hear x not knowing much at all about Syd or my roots has affected me quite a lot. I also felt he shouldn't be forgotten. I wondered what he was like? If I was anything like him? These things are quite normal to want to know, you know! You never told me about your early life."*

She then replied *"Wrote you a very long letter about all you want to know.*

Read it and I think you will understand a lot I have got your address off someone close to me Hope you don't mind x

You will see why you are so fond of music. didn't let you know before did not think you would be interested. Sorry I'm stupid.

Must go now feeling a bit down after going through my useless emotions x"

My mother later responded: *"Neither of us had the education to be parents..."*

And she added.

"I've never wanted to tell you all of this love because it was hard but I'm so sorry your dad didn't have chance to even hold you. Did you like your photo when you were six-month-old you were the only thing I had to live for then, but it was worth it xx

Glad I did not use that bloody gas oven. Never had one since, silly sod that I am x

I was glad she didn't use the gas oven too...

21ST MARCH 12:18

Today is your dad Syd s birthday. It's a long time gone by. But never forgotten I have worried about you since you were a baby wondering if your dad's illness would affect you.

If my mother were alive now I would write this in reply to her last text.

Hi Mum,

Wherever you are.
    I think my dad's illness might finally have caught up with me, however coping well, for now….

Love

Your son

Alan
xxx

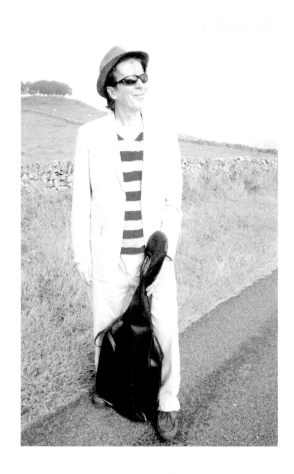

Printed in Great Britain
by Amazon